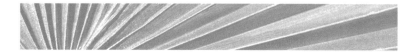

THE
NONI
REVOLUTION

*Today's Tropical Wonder that Can
Battle Disease, Boost Energy and
Revitalize Your Health*

RITA ELKINS, M.H.

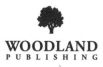

WOODLAND
PUBLISHING

Copyright © 2002 by Rita Elkins

The CIP record for this book is available from the Library of Congress.

For ordering information, contact:
Woodland Publishing, P.O. Box 160, Pleasant Grove, Utah 84062
(800) 777-2665
info@woodlandpublishing.com

The information in this book is for educational purposes only and is not recommended as a means of diagnosing or treating an illness. All matters concerning physical and mental health should be supervised by a health practitioner knowledgeable in treating that particular condition. Neither the publisher nor author directly or indirectly dispenses medical advice, nor do they prescribe any remedies or assume any responsibility for those who choose to treat themselves.

ISBN 1-58054-349-9

Printed in the United States of America

Please visit our website:
www.woodlandpublishing.com

Contents

Acknowledgments

I want to thank Frank and Trudy Kunze, Matrix Health Products, Nutrican Nutritionals, and the International Noni Certification Council, who provided personal accounts of successful noni use. In addition, many thanks to Stephen Center, M.D., for his valuable support. Finally, I would like to express my deep appreciation to Jessica Jones-Sansom for countless hours spent in performing her editing wizardry.

Introduction

We are in the middle of a health revolution. Scientific research into incurable and terminal illnesses is progressing at a promising rate, and conventional treatments for the most common killers—like heart disease, cancer and diabetes—continue to be improved and refined. As consumers, we are inundated with health information on television, in magazines and on the internet. As a result, our consciousness about exercising, eating right, and reducing stress and other health risks has been raised. Furthermore, more people are including treatments outside the mainstream into their health regimen to address their chronic and acute problems, especially those issues that have not been answered by conventional medicine. In fact, according to a 2001 report from the *Annals of Internal Medicine*, two-thirds of Americans have tried some kind of alternative therapy. And many treatments once labeled as "alternative"—like chiropractic therapy, acupuncture and yoga—are gradually gaining acceptance from the medical community as research into these methods lends them more credibility.

Notwithstanding all of this and despite our many successes, there is definitely room for improvement. The number of obese Americans continues to grow, despite the availability of gyms and diet foods. Approximately 60 percent of adults are overweight or obese as are almost 13 percent of children. Furthermore, the number of Americans with (often) preventable diseases, such as type-2 diabetes and heart disease, is on the rise. Currently, about 300,000 people die each year from illnesses related to being overweight, and many of us suffer from nutrient deficiencies even though we have year-round access to a wide variety of healthy foods. The truth is, while we are gaining ground in some health arenas, we are losing ground in others. These failures, however, aren't inevitable. The resources we need to stay informed about our health are out there, as are the means to get and stay healthy, but collectively, we are still falling short.

Why? There is no simple answer. I believe part of the problem deals with our failure to make proper use of our resources—often out of a lack of awareness or because we do not know how. This is compounded by the fact that we receive plenty of contradictory health information (and even misinformation) from the media. In addition, many of us are not serious about getting healthy or our lifestyles do not support healthy living. We are encouraged to spend more and more time at work, and we eat on the run. Some of us sit in front of a computer for hours at a time and spend the little free time we have in front of the television eating processed junk foods. And we take antacids, sleeping pills and antidepressants to mask the inevitable side effects of such a lifestyle. But there is hope.

The best way to achieve and maintain good health is by developing a whole-health strategy, which includes regular exercise, a good diet, and overall healthy living. Complementary and alternative medicine (CAM) may offer you additional help in achieving your health goals, whether you use it as a substitute for a conventional remedy or in conjunction with mainstream medicine. Hawaiian *Morinda citrifolia* (noni) is one multi-purpose CAM treatment that has received considerable attention—both good and bad—in recent years, which brings me to the topic of this book.

Maybe you picked up *The Noni Revolution* because you have already heard of noni or are currently using it but want to learn more about what it does and how to use it for maximum benefit. Or perhaps you've never heard of noni and are curious about it because you want to improve your health. Or, you may be skeptical about the claims that are made about noni by supplement companies and want to see the data supporting these so-called health benefits.

If any of these scenarios apply to you, whether you are new to the world of complementary and alternative medicine (CAM) or a long-time user of CAM treatments like noni, this book is for you. Even with our easy access to unlimited health information (via the internet, etc.), it is often still difficult to separate fact from fiction, especially when you have questions about natural medicine. Finding accurate information on treatments outside the mainstream can be frustrating and time consuming. There are thousands of sites claiming to have new and objective noni information, and several books and pamphlets that have been published about noni.

While doing my own research on noni, however, I was surprised by how much noni information was supplied by companies distributing noni for profit. Many noni claims were supported solely by subjective testimonials and not by science, making some noni users seem more like members of an exclusive club.

In fact, many web and print sources I examined made outrageous claims about what noni could do. Because of exaggerations and distorted information about noni's potential, it has been discredited by many healthcare professionals and rejected as a mainstream treatment. This is not surprising considering that in recent years, there has been a backlash against trends in alternative medicine. Remember the ephedra scare? Current apprehensions about natural medicine are meant to prompt further research into the correct use and safety information on CAM treatments. Not all alternative treatments are safe or effective, people are discovering. As ineffective or dangerous treatments are uncovered, CAM proponents and consumers become more cautious about what methods they advocate and use.

An unfortunate side effect of all of this is that some herbs and other treatments are automatically dismissed. Many scientists and doctors assume that noni has no merit, and their minds are closed. Frequently, noni has been judged before all the evidence has come in, when in fact, initial studies suggest that noni has real health possibilities.

Consider this: What if the same methods used by the scientific community to "evaluate" noni and other alternative therapies were used to determine the benefits of traditional pharmaceuticals? How many effective treatments for cancer, diabetes or depression never would have been discovered? Although it is better to err on the side of caution, the medical community often shows selective concern—being overly critical of certain kinds of treatments while ignoring the risks of others. How else can one explain the Fen-Phen disaster?

The backlash against the CAM health movement has given rise to collective skepticism. Noni critics call it nothing more than "snake oil" peddled by money-hungry supplement companies—false hope in a bottle. And their concern is real. For a variety of reasons, many alternative treatments do not deliver on their promises. After doing research on noni for this book, however, I can honestly say that I don't believe noni is one of those treatments. In order to alleviate some of your concerns about noni, let me briefly respond to some of the common arguments against it:

• *The benefits of noni can't be proven. Supporters rely on testimonials and insufficient research, or they take valid scientific research and manipulate it to "prove" their unsubstantiated claims.*

Actually, there is promising research being done on noni that is being reported in journals like *Phytotherapy Research*, *Cancer Research* and *AIDS Patient Care and STDs*. There are currently more than a dozen studies about noni in print, and subsequent research is and will certainly be done in the future as more of its benefits are uncovered. Researchers in Germany, France, Canada and Austria have investigated noni, and several studies on noni constituents have emerged from the University of Hawaii and at the National Academy of Sciences.

Scientists are also finding connections between noni research and current scientific research in other related areas. For instance, ursolic acid, one compound found in noni leaf, has recently been classified as a natural chemopreventive agent. Scientific trials have confirmed that this powerful acid was able to inhibit a number of cellular changes in human breast cells that can cause the growth of cancerous tumors. And a 2000 issue of the *International Journal of Oncology* investigated the effect of ursolic acid on the growth of human prostate cells and found that this acid promoted the death of potentially malignant cells. In other words, ursolic acid helped to program cancer cells to self-destruct.

It is also true that anecdotal evidence comprises a large part of the support for noni at this writing. Although this evidence on its own is not enough to give noni or any other CAM treatment credibility, it definitely has its place. Often, word of mouth is how products like noni first get noticed since they don't have the money backing that pharmaceutical companies do. If enough people, however, benefit from a product and talk about it, it will eventually get the attention and financial support it needs to be properly researched and tested. And when scientific evidence is added to existing anecdotal evidence, proof of noni's potential becomes even more solid. It just takes a while for research to catch up, to provide exact answers to why and how noni works.

• *Just the fact that noni is a traditional remedy does not mean that it is a valid remedy.*

It is true that no one should classify noni as a bona fide

healing agent just because it qualifies as a traditional folk remedy. It is also true that its long history of use, combined with current research and anecdotal evidence supporting it, lends some credibility to noni. In fact, many traditional remedies that were dismissed with the advancement of mainstream medicine are currently being rediscovered. Of course, not all traditional treatments are effective for the scores of ailments that they may have been originally used for; still, there are a number of cases where traditional remedies do have merit, i.e. St. John's wort, ginkgo, ginseng, saw palmetto, etc.

• *There is an astonishing lack of support for noni from the scientific community and the FDA.*
To say there is a conspiracy by drug companies and the medical community against CAM medicine would be an exaggeration, but money, bureaucracy and politics do factor into what is made available to you—and what isn't—when you visit your doctor, your pharmacist or your local drugstore. Although mainstream medicine is indispensable, other methods outside of the narrow construct of "legitimate" healthcare can be very helpful. Unfortunately, they have a harder time getting noticed and endorsed by the medical community for reasons that will be explained in more detail later in this book. The short answer as to why these oversights happen is a combination of apprehension about nontraditional medicine and a lack of funding.

Furthermore, the FDA currently has no jurisdiction over supplements like noni as long as there are no health claims made on its packaging. This is because natural compounds are not categorized as drugs, but rather as "dietary supplements" and can only be investigated by the FDA in cases where there has been a reported injury or complaint. Their limited power in regulating complementary and alternative medicine and establishing its efficacy and safety does present problems. Although the National Institute of Health and the Office of

Alternative Medicine are trying to address such issues, until a workable plan is initiated, the FDA's opinions on supplements like noni have to be taken with a grain of salt.

• How can I take noni seriously when multi-level marketing is involved?

Although "multi-level marketing" has become a dirty word of sorts, noni should not be discounted based on its method of distribution by some companies (it should also be noted that noni can be found in retail stores as well). Earlier I mentioned the vast difference between the money available to drug companies for research, production and marketing compared with supplement companies. In fact, pharmaceutical companies spent over two billion dollars on advertising to the public—in the year 2000 alone. In 1998, the total advertising budget for the allergy drug Claritin *exceeded the annual budget for Coca Cola* ($185 million compared with $154 million). Supplement companies that sell noni (and other) products do not have that kind of money (or other backing) at their disposal and often start as "grass roots" organizations that use other methods to get the word out about their products. They rely on word of mouth and good products to succeed. And succeed they have.

• Noni's benefits are exaggerated. How can one thing cure so many diseases?

Critics of noni often dismiss it as a fraud because it is used to treat multiple ailments. They compare noni to traditional pharmaceuticals, which are often targeted to treat one illness. This is an unfair comparison since noni contains numerous agents with various healing properties, as do most natural health products. For instance, noni's analgesic and anti-inflammatory properties not only make it effective for joint and muscle pain, but for headaches and earaches and tooth pain as well. Noni's effect on blood flow makes it effective for preventing clotting, stroke, high blood pressure and heart disease, and its antimicrobial constituents are useful to treat colds and flu, staph infections and gingivitis.

Other herbs and supplements also treat multiple ailments. Ginger has been found to be effective for motion and morning sickness, but it also treats bronchitis and rheumatic complaints. Or what about a more common supplement—magnesium? This mineral is often prescribed for depression, PMS, fibromyalgia, cardiovascular problems and tooth decay. Noni has a broad range of health-promoting effects due to, at least in part, its positive effects on basic cell function and its ability to enhance immunity.

Furthermore, there are prescription drugs that are also used to treat varying problems. Consider Sarafem, targeted to treat a premenstrual disorder called premenstrual dysphoric disorder (PMDD), which is characterized by anxiety, irritability, marked depression, mood swings and decreased activity. The active ingredient in this drug is the same active ingredient in the antidepressant Prozac, which has also been prescribed to treat fibromyalgia. And this is just one of many examples of cross-treating with the same medication.

Granted, noni is not a cure-all or a "magic bullet" for disease. It is true, however, that we do not yet know the full extent of what noni can and cannot do. What we do know is that there is more than enough evidence supporting noni use to treat disease and promote health. This book can show you how to do just that. *No matter what your current health strategy is—traditional or alternative—noni can complement your current methods and may improve your quality of life.* It may even inspire you to improve your health in other ways and eradicate bad health habits.

With well over a billion dollars in sales over the last five years, consumer interest in noni is yet to peak. According to *Supplement Industry Executive*, noni sales went up more than

1,000 percent in the twelve months ending in July 2001—an increase that underscores its remarkable rise from obscurity to notoriety over a short period of time. In response to this unprecedented demand, the commercial cultivation of noni has skyrocketed in designated farms located in Tahiti, Tonga and Hawaii. Noni juice sports various product labels and can also be found in chewable tablets, capsules and topical applications. Supplements containing noni leaf and root compounds are also available and have found credibility due to the emergence of studies verifying the therapeutic properties of their chemical constituents. The bottom line—noni has started its own revolution in alternative health. It's here to stay and has rightfully earned its title as a megastar among dietary supplements.

The rest of this book will help you by providing the facts about noni—what it is, where it came from, what it is used for, why it works and current research about noni. I have also included advice on using noni and answer commonly asked questions about noni. To help you even more, I have included a number of side bars with handy information on noni for easy application. Most importantly, this book offers you noni information that is not influenced by noni manufacturers or distributors, but rather is motivated by a desire to provide opportunities for healthier, happier living. Let's take a closer look at why you should consider joining the noni revolution.

CHAPTER ONE

Why Noni?

- Back to the future
- The "health in a pill" mentality
- Treat the whole body, not just symptoms
- Change is slow in coming, but it is coming
- The era of the "syndrome"
- What is CAM?
- Integrative medicine: the best of both worlds
- Why noni?
- The truth about alternative medicine: what you can and can't expect
- Morinda citrifolia: part of a whole-health strategy

Do you suffer from chronic stress or pain? How about persistent fatigue or insomnia? Do you regularly get sinus, ear or bladder infections? Or are you at risk for heart disease, diabetes or any other serious illness? If so, you are not alone. Many Americans suffer from chronic health problems—too many. Everything has a price, and despite the many perks that come with modern living, mainstream American lifestyle has its costs too—like heart disease, obesity and depression, just to name a few. High-stress living, lack of exercise, poor diet and numerous other bad habits that we "just don't seem to have the time to change" are more deadly than you might think. Consider the following statistics:

- There are currently sixteen million diabetics in the United States. Each day approximately 2,200 people are diagnosed with diabetes, accounting for 798,000 new cases reported to the American Diabetes Association in 2001. The most common form of diabetes, type-2 or adult onset, accounts for *over 90 percent* of all cases. The American Diabetes Association says that this type of diabetes is "nearing epidemic proportions, due to an increased number of older Americans, and a greater prevalence of obesity and sedentary lifestyles."

• According to 2002 statistics from the American Cancer Society, men in the U.S. have a little less than one in two lifetime risk of developing cancer; women have a little less than one in three risk. The 2002 edition of *Cancer Facts and Figures* estimates that about one-third of the over half a million cancer deaths expected this year will be related to poor nutrition, lack of exercise, obesity and other lifestyle factors.

• Since 1900, cardiovascular disease (CVD) has been the number one killer in the United States every year except 1918. In 1999, CVD claimed nearly a million American lives accounting for one of every 2.5 deaths that year. According to the American Heart Association's 2002 *Heart and Stroke Statistical Update*, over sixty million Americans currently have one or more types of CVD; over fifty million have high blood pressure. Despite hereditary factors, both high blood pressure and CVD are largely preventable with regular exercise, a nutritious diet and overall healthy living.

• It is estimated that the annual cost of chronic pain in America, including medical expenses, lost income, lost productivity, compensation and legal charges, is close to fifty billion dollars. Furthermore, prescription pain killer use has tripled to over $1.8 billion since 1996. Although a study in *The New England Journal of Medicine* estimated the risk of prescription narcotic addiction to be about one in 3,000, this figure does not take into account at risk groups or those with a history of addiction. According to a recent report from the Surgeon General, middle-class women and older individuals are most at risk, and these groups are the primary users of pain medication and sedatives. Others at risk are those that misuse drugs—including overuse, underuse and erratic use.

BACK TO THE FUTURE

Modern technology has changed the way we eat and the quality and types of foods we eat. It has also influenced the way we live, the environment we occupy, and as a result, the vigor of our lives. There are toxins in the air we breathe, the water we drink and the soil in which we grow our food. Many aspects of modern living considered "normal" (the consumption of alcohol, sugar and fast food for instance) may also have toxic effects on our bodies. The consequences of stress, exposure to harmful toxins, our dietary and exercise habits and our dependence on pharmaceuticals to survive has caused a health epidemic. In response to these and other "side effects" of living in the twenty-first century, scientists and doctors have discovered new ways to treat emerging and existing health problems. Now more than ever, we need better strategies to counteract the negative effects of modern living. Using medicinal plants like noni is one of those strategies.

Over the years, we have made extraordinary advances in the field of medicine. From the first insights about human anatomy and the discovery of penicillin to the first heart transplant and recent progress in cancer treatment, the medical community has found ways to improve health and increase longevity. Medical doctors and researchers have played a huge role in improving the quality and quantity of our lives. Still, many are now discovering that mainstream medicine does not always provide the best options for complete treatment, especially for some chronic illnesses.

THE "HEALTH IN A PILL" MENTALITY

We live in a society that is quick to medicate itself without examining the "whys" of disease. Wanting a cure-all in the form of a pill isn't a new concept. Opiates have been used for pain relief and to create a sense of well-being since Sumerian times. And as recently as the 1800s, heroin was an ingredient in Bayer aspirin until its addictive side effects were better understood. Now more than ever, we look to a pill as the answer to virtually any potential health problem, whether physical or mental. Viagra, for instance, has generated sales of about one billion annually and has over eight million users worldwide. And until generic forms of Prozac were approved, the drug's maker, Eli Lilly & Company, was generating over two billion in annual sales.

Our houses are flooded with television commercials and magazine ads touting the healing powers of scores of "wonder drugs." In fact, in 1997, the FDA eased restrictions on the advertising of prescription drugs, allowing the U.S. to become the first (industrialized) nation to allow "direct-to-consumer" advertising for drugs. Whether it is worry, anxiety, depression, PMS, obesity, arthritis or acne, all of these ads promise that life can return to "normal"—except for the seizures, insomnia or my favorite, "sexual side effects"—if you just pop a pill. Plus, you can treat the side effects of your miracle pill with another pill.

TREAT THE WHOLE BODY, NOT JUST SYMPTOMS

The fundamental flaw in this line of thinking is the idea that the way to "fix" health problems is to treat symptoms. Masking the symptoms of a disease by relying on pills does not get rid of it; it simply helps you "deal" with it. The way to achieve true health requires more than that—it requires that you find the cause of sickness and base treatment on causes rather than symptoms. For instance, taking an aspirin doesn't rebuild your joints or unclog your arteries, but aspirin is recommended for treating arthritis and preventing heart attacks. And aspirin comes with its own set of side effects, including easy bruising, stomach aches, ulcers and gastrointestinal bleeding. But if you were to exercise, eat healthy and take the supplements your bones and heart need to function at optimal levels, you could prevent arthritis or heart disease in the first place thereby avoiding the symptoms altogether.

CHANGE IS SLOW IN COMING, BUT IT IS COMING

A medical mindset persists among some doctors that emphasizes a reliance on drugs over any other alternative: sleeping pills for insomnia, prozac for depression and antibiotics for acne. The truth is, the medical community, despite appearances, is a very conservative body that is slow to change. Even in areas of healthcare research endorsed by mainstream medicine, there are often decades between the discovery of an idea and its implementation, and when it comes to nontraditional care, some in the community would prefer that these treatments remained forever in limbo.

Why? Some of the skepticism and hesitancy is simply due to caution and a desire for thorough research to ensure safety and effectiveness. On the other hand, all to often, some medical professionals refuse to relinquish their previous beliefs in favor of new ideas and better ways of thinking. Other ideas simply do not conform with traditional methodologies and are difficult to test in the "right" way—meaning "objective" and quantifiable double-blind, randomized research trials.

The truth of this is particularly evident in traditional treatments for chronic or unexplainable illnesses.

THE ERA OF THE "SYNDROME"

It seems like there is a syndrome or disorder for everything—irritable bowel syndrome, chronic fatigue syndrome, fibromyalgia syndrome, attention deficit disorder, premenstrual dysphoric disorder. In fact, many of these conditions share many symptoms, which has caused some experts to believe that such diagnoses are made prematurely and are counterproductive. In many cases, there is a tendency to diagnose these chronic, "unexplainable" symptoms before enough is known about them. Once labeled as "garbage dump" diagnoses, they become a wasteland for countless generalized or vague symptoms with unknown causes. Hence, finding a cure becomes more difficult (or put on the back burner). Instead, sufferers are put on a drug protocol for maintenance of their condition, not reversal.

One big reason I believe so many people are turning to CAM treatments is the rise of the "syndrome." Those suffering with chronic pain, insomnia, fatigue or gastrointestinal upset are tired of not getting answers from their doctors. Some suffer more side effects from the drugs prescribed to treat their problems than from the problems themselves. Others get to the point where they take matters into their own hands, refusing to accept the notion that their condition is incurable. One of the greatest benefits of using natural medicine is that it empowers you to take responsibility for your own treatment. Natural medicine is appealing because at the core of its philosophy is the belief that nature provides us with just about everything we need to get healthy. Unlike conventional medicine, which works from the outside in, natural remedies like noni heal from the inside out.

The Pain Plague

Pain. It's just a part of life, right? It's the body's way of telling you that something is wrong. But what happens when the pain doesn't go away? Chronic and unexplainable pain—back pain, neck pain, joint pain and headache pain—is the subject of a growing body of research written about in books and talked about on shows like Oprah and the Today Show. It seems like every day there is a new "cure" for chronic pain. Nevertheless, it remains the top reason for disability, surpassing heart disease and cancer, and it is one of the top three reasons for doctor visits.

Twenty million Americans suffer with chronic pain for at least half of each year. One can't help but wonder why, in a high tech medical era, the number of chronic pain sufferers continues to grow. The increase could be the result of our stressful and sedentary lifestyles, or the fact that people are living longer and more are surviving degenerative diseases. (Individuals over forty-five and those with a history of diseases or accidents are more prone to chronic pain.)

What can we do about it? The healthcare community's answer to chronic pain is medication, despite an unfortunate side effect to this treatment: addiction. Pain killer addiction is not a new problem but is troubling nonetheless. And for those not addicted, there are other serious side effects, including depression, insomnia, kidney or liver damage, stroke, nausea or vomiting, ulcers, memory loss, anxiety, high blood pressure and heart disease. However, proponents of complementary medicine believe there are alternatives to medication for the treatment of chronic pain. Noni is one effective alternative to pain medication.

WHAT IS CAM?

Complementary and alternative medicine (CAM) encompasses healthcare practices that are not currently an integral part of conventional medicine. What is considered CAM is continually changing as CAM therapies are proven safe and effective and become accepted into mainstream medicine. It is estimated that, worldwide, only 10 to 30 percent of people use conventional medicine, compared with *between 70 and 90 percent* who use complementary and alternative medicine.

CAM treatments include a wide variety of systems and methodologies. For instance, whole medical systems (i.e. Ayurvedic medicine, homeopathic medicine) can be described as complementary medicine, as can individual treatments with herbs or supplements like noni (also called "biologically-based treatments"), mind-body treatments like meditation and biofeedback, and "body-based" methods like therapeutic massage and osteopathic manipulation. Energy therapies such as those that use magnets or electromagnetic fields are also part of the CAM definition. Despite the variety in treatment types and styles, the tried and true philosophy of natural healing remains the same:

- Do no harm to the patient.
- Identify and treat the cause of disease, not just its symptoms.
- Promote the role of physician as teacher as well as healer.
- Work with the healing power of nature, not against it.

INTEGRATIVE MEDICINE: THE BEST OF BOTH WORLDS

The numerous advantages of these philosophical tenets are clear. Treatments often have fewer side effects, and they work with the body (instead of in spite of it). They also treat the body as a whole; Western medicine considers each body system to be self-contained. Most of all, CAM offers some a permanent solution for health problems considered hopeless or incurable. Multiple factors conspire against optimal care using the conventional healthcare system today, especially for chronic illnesses: politics, insurance complications, cutting costs and the allure of the almighty dollar often interfere. Luckily, CAM practitioners are often more accepting than some conventional doctors, and encourage their patients to make the most of both conventional and alternative treatments.

In fact, this kind of "integrative medicine" is slowly gaining a following among traditional doctors as well, especially in the treatment of cancer and related illnesses where mainstream options fall short. According to CNN, about one-half of all medical schools offer courses in alternative medicine—about one-third in America, including Harvard, Yale, Johns Hopkins and Georgetown. Furthermore, the American Medical Association (AMA) encourages its members to be better informed about CAM therapies.

By combining the best of mainstream and natural medicine, individuals have more opportunity for greater health. To demonstrate, consider the following scenario: A woman is diagnosed with the early stages of breast cancer. Her medical doctor recommends surgery and chemotherapy for treatment. These options would help to remove the cancer threat, but would unfortunately leave her vulnerable to future illness due to the toll they take on her body's natural defenses. A naturopathic doctor, on the other hand, might offer a diet and supplement regimen to boost her immune system, so her body would be more prepared to fight off the cancer or its recurrence. Granted, this regimen may not offer her as much success without first removing the tumor. The point is that each option has something beneficial to offer the woman. In other words, by combining treatments, the woman not only has a greater chance of survival, but also of achieving and maintaining good health. She now can fight off the cancer without decimating her natural defenses.

Medicine "Outside the Margins"

According to the World Health Organization (WHO), an estimated three billion people (between 60 and 80 percent of the world's population) rely on alternative medicines, including noni, as their primary form of healthcare. If this is true, why is there still so much resistance from the medical community in the United States? Why do so many American doctors reject integrative medicine?

For those readers who are still apprehensive, consider the differences in the way the U.S. deals with complementary medicine compared with Germany. In Germany, one in three doctor prescriptions is an herb. Germany also has a commission whose job is to regulate botanicals in medicine and contribute funding toward research. If an herb is proven safe and effective, it can be labeled with approved health claims and prescribed for those problems.

Currently, the United States has no such system. Medicinal plants marketed in the United States are considered "dietary supplements," not drugs, and their labels cannot make any health claims without certain kinds of research to back them up. And despite some changes in the government's attitude toward CAM methods, very little funding goes toward research. Due to the method in which herbs are categorized, they cannot be regulated by the FDA. The FDA can only respond to complaints of injury or death related to a supplement.

In 1994, a symposium was held in Washington D.C. to discuss these problems. Delegates from the National Institute of Health (NIH), the Office of Alternative Medicine (OAM), the Herbal Research Association and the FDA met to discuss how to better integrate natural treatments into conventional healthcare. Participants tackled issues such as establishing the safety and effectiveness of herbal treatments as well as discussing how to regulate and classify various herbs. Although

"Noni has impressed me"

"I have used Hawaiian noni for the past six years in my clinical practice for general health enhancement, as well as for a wide variety of medical conditions, including chronic pain, irritable bowel syndrome, fibromyalgia, mood disorders, chronic headaches, fatigue and deficient immune function.

Noni has impressed me with its effectiveness and safety with these and other conditions. My patients report improvement within several days to weeks, including symptoms such as headaches, intestinal hypermotility, muscle and joint pain and stiffness, anxiety, depression and low energy. I recommend noni to patients looking for a versatile herbal approach toward improving their health and wellness."

Stephen A. Center, M.D.
Diplomate, American Academy of Anti-Aging Medicine
Medical Director, Matrix Health Products

participants agreed that natural medicine does have potential use in healthcare, especially in areas of cancer research, they could not resolve how to make alternative methods a credible part of mainstream healthcare. Because natural products cannot be patented, very few manufacturers of botanical medicine can afford to do the rigorous testing required by the FDA for approval.

A Medical Monopoly on Money

It may seem odd that federal funding remains inadequate, especially when you consider that Americans spend billions on unconventional healthcare each year—most of it out of pocket. On the other hand, remember that prescription drug companies are in competition with natural health industries and have more money and influence to control the market. If conventional healthcare industries are so powerful, why are they worried about holistic medicine? Well, consider the fact that in the early '90s statistics showed that Americans were actually making more annual visits to unconventional health-care practitioners than to their doctors. Moreover, some insurance companies have recently made changes in their policies to include coverage for certain CAM treatments.

This may not seem like a big deal to you, but consider the loss in profits if, for instance, the primary treatment for back pain was acupuncture instead of pain killers? Or what if Prozac lost its position as the main treatment for depression? Of course, conventional medicine will probably never become obsolete, at least not in the near future, but it doesn't take much competition to threaten profits. The resistance from the medical community to CAM methods like noni has to be taken with a grain of salt. Ultimately, the best way to find out if natural medicine will work for you is to try it for yourself.

WHY NONI?

When you consider all of the natural options available for contemporary healthcare, you can't help but wonder, why noni? What does noni have to offer that other more "proven" conventional and alternative methods can't give you? These questions will be answered in more detail in the next chapter and throughout the rest of the book. Let me give you a brief overview now of why I believe noni should be viewed as an essential supplement in almost every health strategy.

One of the most exciting aspects of noni is its versatility for a variety of conditions. Current and historical use of noni supports its use for a broad range of complaints. Noni is not a cure-all by any means, but it has a broad range of nutrients and therapeutically active substances that have multiple medical uses.

One important chemical that may be at the heart of noni's medicinal value is called xeronine. This substance is believed to help cells function properly. Without it, cells would not be able to carry out the specific responsibilities they were designed for. Cell malfunction is not only linked to cancer, but also arthritis, diabetes and numerous other health problems. If xeronine has the ability to encourage correct cell function, it is easy to see how the xeronine-enhancing properties in noni could have positive effects on a number of illnesses, especially those where faulty cells are a factor. This is just one of the many health-promoting actions attributed to noni—over fifty have been identified so far.

In fact, the noni plant is such a complete source of nutrition that for centuries it was utilized as a source of nourishment in times of famine. Below are just a few of the health problems that may be relieved by using noni:

- chronic pain and arthritic symptoms
- low energy levels; fatigue
- obesity
- high blood pressure
- diabetes
- weak immune system
- cancer

The Medicine with a Brain

Noni is a classic example of an adaptogenic herb. The term "adaptogen" refers to any substance that increases the body's resistance to stress or disease. Noni contains naturally occurring vitamins, minerals, trace elements and co-factors. Moreover, every portion of the noni plant contains a rich array of natural chemicals with desirable effects on the body. There is no pharmaceutical agent that can offer the same benefits. In addition, the beauty of botanical medicines is that they are intuitive about what your body needs. In other words, they adapt to whatever your individual health needs are. Although noni is not the only medicinal plant with multiple uses, its potential health contributions are unique and valuable. Anyone interested in achieving long-term health should consider supplementing with noni.

THE TRUTH ABOUT ALTERNATIVE MEDICINE: WHAT YOU CAN AND CAN'T EXPECT

Once you decide to try alternative medicine, you may get some flak from your doctor, and maybe even friends and family, but you aren't alone. One in three Americans have used alternative medicine and more than 80 percent said they would use it again. Your experience with natural medicine can be pleasant if you know what to expect and you stay informed, especially if you are using products like noni that force more discussion on a controversial subject.

For instance, one big reason that many people trust prescription drugs over natural supplements is because they are approved by the FDA and so they are assumed to be safe. The real question is what exactly does "approved" mean? Although prescription medications must be tested before they can be marketed, this does not ensure their safety. Remember Fen-Phen? Advertisements for drugs may downplay the side effects, but that does not make them any less real. Getting FDA-approved is beneficial, but it is not a fail-safe process.

Furthermore, many doctors prescribe approved drugs for "off-label" purposes—as many as five out of every ten prescriptions. This means that up to one-half of all prescriptions in the U.S. are being taken for purposes other than those they were FDA approved for. Ultimately, many prescribed medicines are no more substantiated than CAM alternatives, and

Comparing CAM with Mainstream Medicine

Mainstream	Complementary
considers the body in parts	considers the body a whole
body and mind separate	body and mind linked
treats the symptoms	treats the causes of illness
attempts to cure disease	tries to prevent disease
uses drugs and surgery	addresses diet and lifestyle
physicians must be detached	caring is vital to healing
physician has sole control of treatment	patient is intimately involved in treatment

most CAM treatments have fewer side effects and are far safer if used correctly for the right ailments. Equally important is the fact that just because a treatment is considered "natural" does not mean it is harmless. As with any medical treatment, alternative therapies like noni supplementation must be undertaken with care. Below are some tips to help you safely use complementary medicine for maximum benefit:

• Alternative treatments are no more of a "magic bullet" than conventional medicine. No one treatment can cure everything. Keep your expectations reasonable, and do not believe anyone who tells you one treatment can cure every problem.
• More is not always better. Follow recommended dosages unless advised otherwise by your doctor. Some supplements are toxic in high dosages. Others may render the opposite of the desired effect if you take too much. For example, optimal zinc supplementation boosts your immune system, but too much of it is immunosuppressive.

- Although certain herbs work better when combined, it is usually not a good idea to take every suggested herb or supplement for a particular health problem. Why take ten supplements when one or two will do? Also, it is harder to tell which herb or herb combination is giving you the most benefit when you are supplementing with dozens of herbs at once. It will be easier on your wallet if you can find a couple of supplements that work effectively.
- Have patience. The effects of herbal treatments are more subtle than prescription drugs and have a cumulative effect over time. Most treatments take between one and three months before the effects become obvious.
- Check for drug interactions before taking a supplement, especially if you have a serious illness like diabetes, cancer or AIDS. Some common herbs will interfere with drug treatments or with other supplements.
- Some herbs are not recommended for those with certain health problems, like high blood pressure or liver disorders. If you are pregnant or nursing, you should also be careful. Before beginning any treatment, make sure it will not negatively effect any existing health conditions.
- Don't underestimate the benefits of getting help from a professional. If you are not sure about what to take or how much, schedule a visit with a naturopathic doctor or other expert. Even if you don't see a doctor, be sure to do adequate research before starting a CAM treatment. Valid sources of herbal information can be difficult to determine, especially online. Look at the author's credentials. Did the information come from scientific studies or approved research organizations? Is the information provided by a company selling herbal products? If so, it may not be accurate. The resource section of this book will give you a place to start.
- Most CAM therapies work best when combined with a healthy lifestyle. Regular exercise and a healthy diet are very important, as is stress management.

MORINDA CITRIFOLIA: PART OF A
WHOLE-HEALTH STRATEGY

The best way to get and maintain optimal health is through a combination of traditional and holistic methods, including proper diet, exercise routines, supplements and adequate psychological support. To prevent disease, a person must be viewed and treated as a whole, not in parts. *Morinda citrifolia* is a dietary supplement that can enhance health on its own, but its effects are even more profound when it is part of a complete strategy that considers mind, body and spirit. Here are some basic habits that you may include in your health strategy. These and other strategies will be discussed in more detail throughout the book:

Eat healthy. Reduce your fat, sugar, caffeine and alcohol intake. Eat plenty of fruits, vegetables and whole grains. Replace processed foods with whole foods. Watch portion size and choose healthy snacks like nuts, seeds and fresh produce. Use monosaturated fats like olive oil and try to take flaxseed oil on a regular basis.

Exercise. Walk or do some other aerobic activity at least thirty minutes a day, four to six days a week. Supplement this activity with stretches and strength training two to three days a week. Always consult a doctor before starting any exercise program.

Acquire healthy habits. If you smoke, do whatever it takes to stop. If you suffer from chronic stress, consider doing yoga, meditation or controlled breathing to relax. Chronic stress can aggravate diabetes, PMS, heart conditions and chronic pain, among other things. Also, try to adopt healthy sleeping habits. Go to bed at the same time every evening, and get up at the same time in the morning when possible.

Take a multi vitamin/mineral supplement. Even if you choose not to take any other herb or supplement besides noni, you should include a multi supplement in your daily routine. Additional supplements will be recommended throughout the book for specific health problems.

Don't forget to detox. Doing some sort of detoxification program every six months to a year is usually a good idea. You can either get guidance from a professional or at a spa, or you can detox on your own with the help of books and other resources on the subject. Consult a doctor about any possible health risks.

Make an appointment to get a physical at least once every year.

Now let's look at noni in more detail, including how it has been traditionally used and current research into its healing compounds and therapeutic applications.

CHAPTER TWO

All About Noni: The Inside Story

Over the last several years, noni fruit (*Morinda citrifolia*) supplementation has spawned a great deal of excitement (and debate) in the United States and abroad. Although some may call this dietary supplement "over-hyped," the noni plant ranks high among historically used therapeutic botanicals because it is so versatile. Rich in alkaloids, terpenes and other health-promoting substances, all parts of the plant have substantial pharmaceutical properties. Its extensive use around the globe gives it further credibility as a valuable herbal medicine. What the peoples of the South Pacific have known and practiced for generations is being scientifically supported today. Clearly, noni has emerged as a botanical that can contribute to our search for health and longevity.

NONI FACTS AT A GLANCE

Scientific Name: Morinda citrifolia

Common Names: Indian mulberry (India), nonu (Samoa and Tonga), nono (Tahiti and Raratonga), Polynesian bush fruit, painkiller tree (Caribbean islands), lada (Guam), mengkudo (Malaysia), nhau (Southeast Asia), grand morinda (Vietnam), cheesefruit (Australia), kura (Fiji), bumbo (Africa)

Parts Used: bark, leaves, flowers, fruit, roots and seeds

Physical Description: Noni is technically an evergreen shrub or small tree with rigid, coarse branches covered with dark, oval, glossy leaves, which can grow as much as twenty feet high. Small, white, fragrant flowers bloom out of its clustered pods. The fruit of the shrub is initially green, turns yellow, and finally creamy-white in color. It is fleshy and gel-like when ripened, resembling a small breadfruit or potato. The flesh of the fruit is characteristically bitter and when completely ripe, produces a very distinctive, somewhat offensive, odor. The shrub can grow to heights of twenty feet and produces buoyant seeds that can float for months in ocean bodies, allowing it to distribute itself on multiple sea coasts great distances apart.

Noni comes from the Rubiaceae family which contains approximately eighty species, twenty of which have economic or other benefits. Noni stands out among its other family members because of its diverse uses and its resiliency. It is able to grow in distinctly different environments, including sandy areas, fertile soils and rocky terrains.

Where Found: Noni is found in most of the islands of the South Pacific, Malaysia, the West Indies, Indonesia, the

Philippines, Taiwan, Vietnam, India, Africa, Australia and Guam.

Characteristics: analgesic, antibacterial, anticongestive, anti-inflammatory, antioxidant, astringent, blood purifier, laxative, lowers high blood pressure, promotes healthy menstrual flow, sedative, softens skin, tonic

NONI PAST AND PRESENT: THERAPEUTIC APPLICATIONS

Below is a summary of traditional and contemporary uses for *Morinda citrifolia*:

abnormal menstruation	abscesses*
acne/boils	afterbirth*
arthritis*	backaches*
blood poisoning	burns/stings*
chronic fatigue syndrome*	colds/flu*
constipation	cough/chest infections*
depression*	diabetes, type-2*
diarrhea*	earaches
eye complaints*	fever*
fibromyalgia	gout
gum disease/soreness*	headaches
heart troubles*	hernias, diaphragmatic*
high blood pressure*	immune weakness*
infections*	insomnia*
intestinal parasites*	jaundice
joint/muscle pain*	liver disease
microbes*	nutrient deficiencies*
pain, acute or chronic*	rheumatism
skin problems*	sore throats*

stomach problems*	stroke*
thrush	thyroid problems*
toothaches*	tuberculosis*
cancerous tumors*	ulcers
urinary disorders*	wounds/fractures*

* Indicates applications currently supported by scientific research

A BRIEF HISTORY OF NONI

Referred to today as the queen of the family Rubiaceae, noni is considered a sacred botanical by the Polynesian people. Although originally found in India and the surrounding regions, noni eventually made its way to the South Pacific. It is believed that immigrants from the Marquesas Islands brought the plant with them to other islands. For over two millennia, island healers utilized every part of the noni plant (leaves, roots, bark, flowers and fruit) to treat a myriad of diseases. Respected and revered for its impressive medicinal power, the ability of the plant to expedite the healing process was so impressive that it was considered magical by island peoples. There is even evidence that ancient Polynesians used noni for clothing dye and food in addition to using it for medicine. It is thought that soldiers stationed on Polynesian islands during World War II were taught by the native Polynesian people to eat Noni fruit to gain endurance and added sustenance.

Common to the unspoiled thickets and forests of Malaysia and Polynesia, and the low hilly regions of the Philippine islands, noni has been cultivated throughout communities in the South Pacific for hundreds of years. The noni tree grows wild in the lush, balmy climates of these islands and can bear fruit continuously, allowing for several harvests throughout the year.

Noni has a long history of medicinal use throughout these areas. It is thought to be the most widely and commonly used medicinal plant prior to the European Era. Noni's use in Hawaii is thought to originate from inter-island canoe travel and settlement dating to before Christ. Its hardy seeds, which have the ability to float, must have also contributed to its distribution among various seacoasts in the South Pacific region.

The plant also has a strong history of use in Tonga, where it grows abundantly. Ancient manuscripts handed down from generation to generation describe many uses for this plant, not the least of which was nutritional. In addition, historical investigation has established the fact that some of Hawaii's earliest settlers probably came via Tahiti. For this reason, Tahitian herbal practices have specific bearing on the herbal therapeutics of islands to the north.

A Source of Sustenance

Cultures familiar with noni not only favored using it for treating diseases, but also utilized it as a source of nourishment in times of famine. Noni fruit has been recognized for centuries as an excellent source of nutrition. So much so, that it was considered a staple food to the people in Tonga, Raratonga, Samoa and Fiji eaten both raw and cooked. The Aboriginal tribes of Australia also consumed the raw fruit flavored with salt. Its seeds, leaves, bark and root were eaten and valued for their individual nutritive and healing properties. While the fruit is an abundant source of enzymes, keep in mind that Noni leaves and roots are considered complete proteins, containing an array of essential amino acids that cannot be produced in the body. Moreover, all parts of the plant offer rich sources of vitamins and minerals including vitamin C, vitamin E, calcium, magnesium and zinc.

A Favorite among Medicine Men

Interestingly, elaborate traditional rituals and praying rites usually accompanied the administration of noni. Clearly, cultures indigenous to these islands had a significant understanding of their native flora. For example, native Hawaiians maintained a folk-medicine taxonomy that was considered second to none. Research indicates that noni was among the few herbal remedies that islanders considered tried and true. In Hawaii, trained herbal practitioners called kahuna laau lapaau reserved the right to prescribe plant therapies. Records indicate that Hawaiian medical practices were based on an extensive and very meticulous description of symptoms. Dosages were controlled and the collection and administration of plant extracts was carefully monitored.

The Hawaii Harvesting Method

The fruit was typically picked before it fully matured (in the yellow stage) and placed in a glass jar in the sunlight. The best time to pick the fruit, according locals, is in the early morning. Then the fruit is left out for five days to a week until the pulp is mushy and juices collect at the bottom of the jar. The juice can then be strained through a piece of cloth into a smaller jar and refrigerated. Some healers picked the unripe noni fruit and ripened it indoors. When it was soft, the fruit was mashed or blended with a little fresh water. It was then forced through a sieve to extract the juice. Noni is cultivated either by seed or cutting.

ANCIENT HEALERS USED THE WHOLE NONI PLANT

It's important to know that folk healers looked to every part of noni to heal and strengthen the body. The leaves and bark stem were pounded and strained, producing a juice prescribed for urinary disorders, swelling and muscle and joint pain. Noni leaf extracts were used to curb excessive blood flow and

Noni Around the World

Australia. Aborigines ate noni fruit as a regular part of their diet.
Burma. Locals use the unripened fruit in their curries, and ate the uncooked ripe fruit with salt. They also roasted the seeds of the fruit.
Fiji. Noni fruit is eaten as a food source either raw or cooked.
Phillipines. Locals used fermented noni fruit to make jam.
Hawaii. Medical practitioners used noni tonics to treat diabetes, stings and burns.
India. The noni fruit is eaten green in curries. Medicinally, Indians used noni to treat fever and gout.
Java. Noni leaves provided a vegetable dish, and their resiliency made them desirable as a fish wrap for cooking.
Nigeria. Noni was used to treat fever, malaria, dysentery and jaundice.
Samoa. Traditionally, noni was used for bowel disorders—especially intestinal parasites, constipation and infant diarrhea, infections, indigestion, skin inflammation, mouth sores, fever, contusions and sprains.
Tahiti. Noni was known for its remarkable ability to purge the intestinal tract and promote colon health. The noni fruit, leaves and bark were also used in the treatment of diabetes, heart troubles and high blood pressure, with different portions prescribed for different illnesses.

discourage the formation of blood clots. The noni leaf was particularly valuable in treating painful joint conditions and in healing inflammatory conditions of the skin. Noni roots had expectorant actions and were used to treat congestion and to shrink swollen membranes. Root compounds also exerted a natural sedative action and lowered blood pressure. Noni's flower essences were employed to relieve eye inflammation.

The most well-known part of noni, the fruit, has a multitude of uses, including the treatment of tuberculosis, arthritis and rheumatism. The juice of the fruit was placed directly on the hair to treat head lice, followed by a rinse of fragrant coconut water. Drinking the juice of the fruit was used to treat painful menstruation, diabetes, gastric ulcers, infection and even depression. The seeds have a purgative action useful for external inflammations and pain.

Even noni bark has therapeutic value. Boiling the astringent bark resulted in decoctions that were administered for wound healing and malaria.

Throughout tropical regions, virtually every portion of the noni bush was used to treat disease or injury and valued for its individual medicinal properties. In relation to its medicinal value, many local healers believed that the fruit was good, but that the leaf and root were even better. In preparing medicinal brews, they almost always used a combination of plant parts for maximum effect. Patoa Tama Benioni, who is a member of the Maori tribe from the Cook Islands and a lecturer on island plants, has stated:

"Traditionally Polynesians use noni for basically everything in the treatment of illness. Noni is a part of our lives. Any Polynesian boy will tell you he's had experience with it. We use juice from its roots, its flowers, and its fruit . . . my grandmother taught me to use Noni from the roots to the leaves to make medicine for external as well as internal use, and for all kinds of ailments, such as coughs, boils, diseases of the skin, and cuts."

Clearly, every part of noni has something to offer us today. Later in the book, we will discuss how to make some of the noni treatments described in this chapter.

NONI PLANT: A SUMMARY OF
PARTS AND USES

Below is a list of traditional and modern uses for noni, listed by plant part. Although not comprehensive, this list should give you a good idea of noni's potential and versatility.

Leaves

Internal—juice of leaves used to treat gout, gingivitis and sties; tea or infusion used to treat fever and blood sugar disorders; sore throats treated by chewing leaves; leaf extracts were used to discourage the formation of blood clots

Topical—pounded leaves for burns, boils and wounds; leaves heated to treat joints and ringworm; leaf poultices used to treat skin abscesses and boils; fresh, crushed leaves rubbed on to treat infant chest colds

The Root

Internal—used traditionally to reduce fever and congestion; root compounds also have a natural sedative quality and can be used to lower blood pressure

Topical—used to treat gout and joint swelling

The Bark

Internal—boiled bark decoctions were given as a drink for stomach ailments, wounds and malaria; dried and powdered bark mixed with water used to treat infant diarrhea

Topical—coughs were treated with grated bark

Flowers

Topical—eyewashes were made from decoctions for eye complaints from flower extracts

The Fruit

Internal—gum and throat problems, dysentery, blood poisoning, abnormal menstrual bleeding, tuberculosis, arthritis, rheumatism, diabetes, high blood pressure, heart troubles, ulcers, infections and as a general tonic and antimicrobial

Topical—poultices of the fruit made with mashed unripe fruit and salt applied to swollen areas, deep wounds, boils, broken bones and inflamed joints; ripe fruit used to treat facial acne, sores and staph infection; juice applied to hair to get rid of lice

Combinations

- A juice made from pounding noni leaves, roots and fruit mixed with water was administered for diarrhea.
- Small pieces of fruit and root infused with water were given to kill intestinal parasites.
- The leaves and stem bark were pounded, strained and drunk as a tonic for joint and muscle pain as well as urinary disorders.

BRINGING NONI TO THIS COUNTRY

Ironically, modern times brought a general lack of interest in the noni plant, until recently. Although some interest in noni developed at the turn of the twentieth century, interest did not continue during subsequent decades when antibiotic drugs and strong synthetic pharmaceuticals were introduced into the medical community. The intrigue generated by the island botanical during the early 1900s diminished until 1950 when an article published in an issue of *Pacific Science* reported that noni fruit possessed significant antibacterial properties, even against the potentially dangerous *E. coli*.

The modern commercialization of noni began in the early 1990s, when individuals from American were introduced to

"I am now getting solid sleep"

"I have been using noni juice for approximately six months now. I started out taking one ounce a day for the first three weeks then increased to two ounces twice a day. In that time, I have noticed an increase in energy and especially in stamina. The noni has been instrumental in clearing up a residual bronchial cough and I have not had bronchitis or a cold since starting it. Another plus (and this one alone is well worth it!) is that for the first time in my life, I am now getting deep, solid sleep. I used to be a very light sleeper and if awakened after the initial four to five hours, would remain awake.

Thanks to noni, that has changed. I'm so pleased! A couple of other benefits I've noticed is that I no longer have shoulder pain in either shoulder—this has also been pretty much a life-long problem; my problems with upset/anger/depression have been somewhat minimized as well—I am more calm! So I'm grateful for noni and hope to have more health benefits in the future."

Olga E.

Hawaiian noni and decided to produce and commercialize it on a mass scale. Morinda, Inc. became one of the first of several companies to bring the health benefits of noni to the international health market.

Noni juice rapidly gained popularity for its medicinal attributes and has been widely marketed throughout the United States and other parts of the world. It's important to keep in mind that while the leaf and root extracts of the noni plant are less well known, their remarkable healing properties are equally valuable. Noni supplements that include other plant parts are also available.

Since noni's international debut, researchers in Germany, France, Canada and Austria have investigated the plant. Several studies on noni's constituents have emerged from the

University of Hawaii and the National Academy of Sciences. As data emerges on its anti-tumor properties, studies have been presented to the American Association for Cancer Research, and articles on noni have appeared in prestigious publications like *Cancer Letter*. We are only beginning to understand the therapeutic and preventive value of this remarkable exotic botanical.

Where is Noni Cultivated Today?

Noni is grown in many Polynesian islands today where the climate is ideal. While Tahiti, Hawaii and the Marquesas Islands of French Polynesia are best known for their noni crop, the island of Tonga and Eua (thought to be the most ancient of the South Pacific isles) offer fertile, virgin soils for its cultivation. In fact, some of the largest organic noni farms are found in Tonga, where the plant has grown wild for generations. The Polynesian Traditional Medicine Council is also located in Tonga and is comprised of a variety of professionals schooled in the use of conventional and ancient medicinals, research and business. Councils like this one strive to study and authenticate the use of traditional medicines of Polynesia. They are also involved in the cultivation of medicinal plants and trees on designated farms for use worldwide. Its members enthusiastically encourage the modern production and application of traditional herbal medicines. They also advocate that these products meet established criteria to determine their Polynesian origin or authenticity.

NONI RESEARCH

Although we will be discussing noni research throughout the book, this section will give you a good introduction into what has been uncovered about noni and its health-promoting benefits. As mentioned earlier, research on noni is still very limited. Noni is the least understood of the five top herbs used in complementary medicine (ginseng, garlic, aloe and lemongrass), according to University of Hawaii medical anthropologist, Nina Etkin, author of *Economic Botany*. This fact may seem damning, but remember that quite a bit of research on natural remedies is done in foreign countries where there is more acceptance of complementary and alternative medicine. This research is often published in foreign journals that are not translated into English. Despite these drawbacks, as more evidence supporting noni is compiled, more research is sure to be done. For the most current research on noni, refer to "Noni Information and Research" section of the **Resource Guide** in the back of this book. Let's look at a few studies that reveal noni's promise in the field of medicine.

THE STUDIES

Anticancer Activity of Ursolic Acid Found in Noni Leaf

One compound found in the noni leaf, called *ursolic acid*, has been classified as a natural chemopreventive agent. Recent scientific trials testing this powerful acid have confirmed its ability to inhibit a number of cellular changes in human breast cells that can cause the growth of cancerous tumors. In these tests, ursolic acid was able to suppress the negative effect of a carcinogenic agent on breast cells. Another currently published study reported that ursolic acid inhibited the growth of a very dangerous form of cancer made up of fibrosarcoma cells. A 2000 issue of the *International Journal of Oncology* investigated the effect of ursolic acid on the growth of human prostate cells and found that this acid promoted the death of potentially malignant cells. In other words, ursolic acid helped to program cancer cells to self-destruct.

Noni Plant Compounds in the Juice and Leaves Boost Immune Function

There is some evidence to support the fact that noni helps to increase T-cell count, the immune cells that fight infections. In this way, noni compounds enable the immune system to function more effectively. The alkaloid and other chemical compounds found in noni have also proven themselves to effectively control more than six types of infectious bacterial strains, including: *Escherichia coli*, *Salmonella typhi* (and other types), *Shigella paradysenteriae*, and *Staphylococcus aureus*. The bioactive components of the whole plant, combined or in separate portions, have demonstrated the ability to inhibit several different microbes. This may explain why noni is commonly used to treat colds and flu.

Alkaloids have been able to boost *phagocytosis*, which is the process in which certain white blood cells attack and literally digest infectious organisms. Interestingly, the anti-tumor action of noni has been ascribed to an immune system response that stimulates T cells. An article published in a 1999 issue of *Phytotherapy* reported that noni fruit contains polysaccharides capable of enhancing immune function. In addition, damnacanthal, found in noni fruit was able to inhibit the early antigen stage of the Epstein-Barr virus, which is involved in diseases like chronic fatigue syndrome and often occurs in people with weak immune function. Moreover, another 1999 study reported that the ursolic acid found in the noni leaf is capable of positively impacting the immune system, which may work to not only discourage the development of cancer, but other viral, bacterial and fungal infections as well. In fact, a 2001 issue of *AIDS Patient Care Studies* found that noni may benefit those with TB.

Diabetes and Noni Leaf Extract

Scientists at the Department of Pharmacology, at the Obafemi Awolowo University, in Nigeria reported in a 1999 issue of the *Journal of Pharmacology* that a leaf extract of *Morinda lucida* had significant hypoglycemic activity in diabetic tests. *Morinda lucida* is a close relative of *Morinda citrifolia*. The glucose-lowering compounds found in this plant suggest a similar chemical composition in noni leaves, which would explain noni's traditional use for blood sugar disorders. Moreover we know that noni leaf contains B-sitosterol, a proven blood sugar lowering compound. In laboratory tests it was able to increase fasting insulin levels and lower fasting glucose levels. By doing so, B-sitosterol offered protection from an excessive rise in blood sugar.

Anti-Inflammatory and Anti-Fever Properties of B-Sitosterol

A study published in *Planta Medica* reported that plant sterols (B-sitosterol in particular) work to reduce inflammation and fever while easing pain. In laboratory tests, researchers concluded that the sterols possess anti-inflammatory properties that rival the steroid drug cortisone and the anti-fever actions of aspirin, and they also worked to reduce swelling. Researchers stressed that these actions occurred with no side effects. They concluded that sterols possess highly potent ant-inflammatory and antipyretic actions with a high margin of safety and should be applied in medical treatment plans. This sheds light on why noni leaf may help with ailments like colds, flu, sore throat, etc. as well as inflammatory conditions.

Cancer and Noni Juice

A 1994 study cited the anticancer activity of noni fruit compounds against lung cancer. A team of scientists from the University of Hawaii used live laboratory mice to test the medicinal properties of the fruit against Lewis lung carcinomas that were artificially transferred to lung tissue. The mice that were left untreated died in nine to twelve days; however, those mice that were given noni juice in consistent daily doses significantly prolonged the life span of the infected mice. Almost half of these mice lived for more than fifty days. Research conclusions stated that the chemical constituents of this juice acted indirectly by enhancing the ability of the immune system to deal with the invading malignancy by boosting macrophage or lymphocyte activity. Further evaluation theorized that the unique chemical constituents of noni fruit enhanced T-cell activity in the immune system, a reaction that may explain the multi-faceted use of noni to treat a variety of infectious diseases. T cells destroy invading microorganisms and abnormal cells.

Damnacanthal: Chemical Compound in Noni May Prevent Malignancies

In Japan, studies on tropical plant extracts found that *damnacanthal*, a compound found in noni fruit was able to inhibit the function of K-RAS-NRK cells, which are considered precursors to certain types of cancerous malignancies. The experiment involved adding noni plant extract to RAS cells and incubating them for a number of days. Observation disclosed that noni was able to significantly inhibit RAS cellular function. Among 500 plant extracts, noni was determined to contain the most effective compounds against RAS cells. Its damnacanthal content was clinically described in 1993 as "a new inhibitor of RAS function." Scientists at the Department of Pharmacology at the John A. Burns School of Medicine in Honolulu also reported in 1996 that the ability of noni juice to modulate or boost the immune system also contributes to its anticancer activity.

Noni Root and Cancer Prevention

In 1999, researchers at the Department of Biochemistry of the School of Medicine at Chiba University in Japan reported that damnacanthal isolated from noni root inhibited an enzyme called *tyrosine kinase*, which helps to promote the growth of malignant cells. Abnormal cells that were treated with the damnacanthal from noni roots prior to exposure to ultraviolet light were more rapidly destroyed. What this study shows is that noni roots constituents can naturally stop the activity of tyrosine kinase. Some of the most powerful chemotherapy drugs we use today to treat cancer have been designed to do the same thing. Noni's damnacanthal content also contributes to programmed malignant cell death. Programmed cell death works to regulate tumor cell growth. In light of this data, damnacanthal from noni may not only prevent cancer, but also be of benefit if you already have cancer.

A 2001 issue of *Cancer Research* also found cancer preventative qualities in two glycosides found in noni juice. The study looked at the effects of the juice on cell transformation in mice with promising results. In fact, the National Institutes of Health (NIH) gave a grant of over 300,000 dollars to Cancer Research Center of Hawaii Doctor Brian Issell in 2001 to test noni in humans because of promising results in other cancer studies using mice. Dr. Issell hopes to uncover more information on the cancer-fighting properties of noni for humans.

Noni Root Extract as a Natural Sleep Aid and Painkiller

French researchers discovered that compounds contained in the root of the noni plant can act as natural pain killers and sedatives and published their findings in a 1990 issue of *Planta Medica*. Using laboratory tests, these scientists discovered that root extracts showed a significant pain-killing action with no toxicity. In addition, they found that the compounds also induced sleep and influenced behavior. They described the effect as "central analgesic activity." Folk use of noni also supports these findings. It has been used for treating both chronic and acute pain conditions.

Anti-Parasitic and Anti-Malarial Action of Morinda Species

In 1999, an article appeared in the December issue of the *Journal of Ethnopharmacology* that singled out leaf extracts from the *Morinda* species, *M. lucida* and *M. morindoides*, for their ability to inhibit parasitic growth in laboratory test studies by over 55 percent. The anthraquinone content of these leaves is what is thought to create a reaction capable of treating malaria and other parasitic diseases as well. The leaves of *M. morindoides* also displayed antiameobic action shedding new light on their traditional application for intestinal infections by ancient medical practitioners. These plant species belong to the same family as *Morinda citrifolia* and share many of the same botanical compounds, including anthraquinones.

Enzymes and Weight Loss

There is also some evidence to suggest that because noni helps to normalize enzymatic functions on a cellular basis, it can help expedite the burning of fat as well as the detoxification of tissue. Enzymes are the catalysts for breaking open a fat cell and using its content for fuel or heat. Noni plant parts are rich in live enzymes, which jump start digestion and provide energy, two functions related to maintaining an ideal weight.

The Solomon Survey

Neil Solomon, M.D., Ph.D., and author of numerous titles on noni, has been conducting research on noni since its initial introduction to Canada and the United States. In the late 1990s, he compiled survey information on noni from data collected from over fifty doctors and 10,000 noni users (some using noni by itself and other combining noni with other treatments). Here is a short summary of some of his findings. For a more complete discussion, refer to his book *The Noni Phenomenon*:

Who's Who in Noni Research

Ralph Heinicke, Ph.D. A pioneer of noni research, Dr. Heinicke remains a prominent figure in new findings about noni. In the 1950s, he was involved in research on pineapples at the Pineapple Research Institute in Hawaii. His research into cancer-fighting pineapple components led him to study related compounds he isolated in noni.

Anne Hirazumi, Ph.D. A biochemist and researcher at the University of Hawaii's Department of Pharmacology, Hirazumi has been an integral part of beginning and continuing various noni research.

Isabelle Abbott, Ph.D. Abbott is an expert botanical scientist who has researched the use of noni for high blood pressure, diabetes and cancer since the early '90s.

- More than two-thirds of the 900 patients taking noni for cancer treatment found that it lessened or reversed symptoms.
- More than half of nearly 1,000 patients who took noni for stroke recovery reported positive results, as well as 80 percent of patients using noni for the symptoms of heart disease. Eight-seven percent said it helped lower high blood pressure.
- Almost 85 percent of the 2,500 type-1 and type-2 diabetics using noni stated that the supplementation improved their condition. Eighty-five percent of those taking noni for chronic pain also experienced relief, including those using it for arthritis and headaches.
- Ninety-one percent of those surveyed experienced increased energy, 71 percent claimed that it helped them deal with

stress better and 72 percent said that they lost weight. Others reported changes in digestion, quality of sleep, mental clarity and symptoms of depression.

AN INTRODUCTION TO NONI'S TOP HEALTH-PROMOTING COMPOUNDS

We are still in the process of discovering exactly how noni works, but as new compounds are identified and understood, the answers to how and why noni functions the way it does are being discovered. Noni contains many health-promoting substances, like vitamins, minerals, enzymes, proteins, that synergistically contribute to its overall effects. While these are invaluable, it is the other less known essential substances in noni that offer profound health benefits. Let's look at a few of them. A more detailed description of these compounds and how they work is discussed in the next chapter:

Xeronine: A substance that is produced by the body and has broad therapeutic power. Xeronine helps healthy cells maintain proper function and abnormal cells regain normal functions. Noni contains high amounts of a substance called proxeronine necessary for the synthesis of xeronine by the body. Only a small amount of proxeronine is produced in the body, so supplementation is beneficial.

Nitric Oxide: Research into the therapeutic benefits of nitric oxide has attracted a lot of attention, especially concerning its effects on high blood pressure. So much so that nitric oxide researchers won the Nobel prize for medicine in 1998. Although noni doesn't contain nitric oxide, it does promote its production by the body. Nitric oxide's effects can be seen in every cellular system.

Ursolic Acid: A compound found in noni that is a natural chemopreventive agent. Ursolic acid helped to program cancer cells to self-destruct. The reasons all of us don't have cancer is that our cells are programmed to "die." In many cancer patients, this safeguard fails to function, thereby allowing the uncontrolled reproduction of cells, hence malignant tumors form. Cancer will be discussed in more detail in a later chapter.

Damnacanthal: Another noni component, damnacanthal, discourages the growth of cancerous tumors. It works on a cellular level to inhibit malignant cell replication. It may be beneficial in the treatment of lung, colon and pancreatic cancers, as well as leukemia.

Scopoletin: First isolated in 1993, this noni component plays an integral role in blood pressure regulation.

THE BOTTOM LINE: NONI'S OVERALL BENEFITS

Today, historical use, research studies and anecdotal surveys support the ability of noni to provide many varied health benefits, from fighting cancer to increasing energy levels. In short, the noni plant has been shown to:

• act as an anti-inflammatory and antihistamine
• help alleviate chronic and acute pain, as well as arthritic symptoms
• inhibit precancerous formations and retard the growth of cancer cells
• promote tissue healing at a molecular level
• act as an antioxidant

- boost energy levels
- reduce high blood pressure
- help regulate diabetes
- exhibit strong antimicrobial properties
- help correct digestive problems and control weight
- enhance immune system cells called macrophages and lymphocytes
- regulates thymocytes (immune cells)

CHAPTER THREE

Inside Noni

- A guide to noni's components
- How does noni work? A closer look at theories on *Morinda Citrifolia*

Now that you have a basic understanding of noni's character and what it is used for, let's explore the mechanisms that give noni its medicinal properties. Looking over the list of health benefits at the end of **Chapter 2**, the complexity of noni emerges. In fact, scientists have identified hundreds of compounds in noni that have both combined and individual healing qualities for a broad range of health problems. Because of its molecular complexity, understanding everything about noni's function in the human body will take more time. Still, the research done so far is promising, and in fact, many of noni's compounds are currently being identified and tested. In the last chapter, I introduced you to some of these compounds and their scientific backing. Now, through a scientific lens, I will give you a more detailed picture of noni and how it ranks as a therapeutic biochemical storehouse.

A GUIDE TO NONI'S COMPONENTS

As mentioned in the previous chapter, the noni plant is rich in health-promoting nutrients and phytochemicals including antioxidants and bioflavonoids. Noni is a classic example of an adaptogenic herb, which increases the body's resistance to stress or disease. Every portion of this plant is endowed with a rich array of natural chemicals capable of initiating desirable actions in the human body. More than 150 isolated compounds have now been identified in the noni plant. You have already been introduced to some of noni's components, but in this chapter, we will look more closely at how they work.

Noni contains an impressive array of alkaloid and terpene compounds. L. asperuloside, aucubin, and glucose have been identified in noni by their acetyl derivatives and both caproic and caprylic acids have been isolated. The alkaloid content of noni fruit and leaves is also thought to be responsible for many of its therapeutic actions. Alkaloids (organic compounds that contain nitrogen) exhibit a wide range of pharmacological and biological activities in the human body. They are also the basis of many medicines. Noni includes or stimulates the production of the following compounds: xeronine, serotonin, damnacanthal, anthraquinones, caratenoids, morindine, sitosterol, glycosides, alizarin, nitric oxide, scopoletin and ursolic acid.

Noni Leaf Pharmacology and Nutrient Profile

The chemical compounds found in noni leaf offer a wide array of natural yet potent pharmaceutical agents as well as an impressive array of amino acids. Amino acids are the building blocks of proteins, and the noni leaf is rich in them, a fact that explains why the leaf is considered a complete source of protein.

Leaf extracts of the noni plant are actually higher in some minerals than the juice. They are also rich in a number of vitamins and minerals and significantly exceed juice levels of phosphorus, iron, calcium, magnesium, vitamin E, vitamin K1 and niacin. In addition, leaf extracts of the plant have a significant amount of protein while the fruit is high in ascorbic acid content. The leaf is also rich in beta-sitosterol, glycosides, ursolic acid and anthraquinones, which are responsible for some of its powerful actions in the human body. Ursolic acid is known to have anti-cancer properties, and B-sitosterol can significantly lower bad cholesterol levels. Noni leaves also contains other compounds that exhibit anti-inflammatory, antibacterial, antiviral and antitumor properties.

Noni Root and Root Bark Pharmacology

The roots of the noni bush are rich in anthraquinones, asperuloside (rubichloric acid), damnacanthal, glycosides, morindadiol, morindine, morindone, sterols, chlororubin, alizarin and other compounds. They are effective for pain relief, to relieve congestion, constipation and to calm the central nervous system. Compounds found in the root have the ability to reduce swollen mucous membrane and lower blood pressure in laboratory studies.

Noni Juice Pharmacology

Proxeronine. Various researchers have speculated that an alkaloid present in noni juice called proxeronine may prompt the production of xeronine in the body. This idea was first proposed by Dr. Ralph M. Heinicke, based on research done at the University of Hawaii. Xeronine, if you remember, is a compound that is produced by the body and is involved in healthy cell regulation. Not only does it help maintain healthy cells, but it also influences abnormal cells so that they may return to normal. Since it works on a cellular level, it beneficially affects every body system.

Proxeronine in noni may signal the body to produce xeronine. Heinicke has theorized that this proenzyme can be effective in initiating a series of beneficial cellular reactions through its involvement with specific proteins. He points out that tissues contain cells with certain receptor sites for xeronine. Mitochondria, microsomes, DNA, RNA, Golgi apparatus and other cell parts are all affected. Because the reactions that can occur are so varied, many different therapeutic actions can result when xeronine production escalates. He believes that this explains why consuming noni juice can be beneficial for so many seemingly unrelated disorders. While we know that noni juice contains powerful enzymes and phytonutrients, the xeronine theory has not yet been completely substantiated by scientific studies, but research done so far does raise some intriguing possibilities for proxeronine.

Damnacanthal. On the other hand, the therapeutic action of this noni fruit compound is backed by scientific data. Damnacanthal has the ability to block or inhibit the cellular function of RAS cells, which are considered pre-cancerous cells. When this occurs, the development of malignant tissue is retarded. Research has shown noni's potent effects on cancerous malignancies, and many believe that damnacanthal is at least partially responsible for noni's cancer-fighting properties. In 1993 research, damnacanthal isolated from noni root (it is found in the fruit and the root) was found to inhibit cancer cell activity by influencing its regulatory signals. Basically, damnacanthal "convinces" cancer cells that they are healthy, which stops or slows cell multiplication and retards cancer growth. This compound may be useful in lung, colon and pancreatic cancer, as well as leukemia.

Scopoletin. This compound was first isolated in noni fruit by researchers at the University of Hawaii in the early 1990s. This early research and later studies on scopoletin confirm its ability to regulate blood pressure. Not only does noni lower high blood pressure, it also raises blood pressure that is below normal. Scientists know that isolated scopoletin can lower blood pressure. When it is used alone, however, without other

What's in Noni?

More than 150 nutraceuticals have been identified in noni so far. Below is a partial list that contains some of the more important health-promoting components of noni based on information from Dr. Anne Hirazumi:

acetic acid	alizarin	alkaloids	anthraquinones
benzoic acid	butanoic acid	calcium	campestrol
carbonate	carotene	cycloartenol	damnacanthal
decanoic acid	elaidic acid	eugenol	ferric iron
glycosides	heptanoic acid	hexadecane	hexanamide
hexose	iron	isobutyric acid	isocaproic acid
isofucosterol	lauric acid	limonene	linoleic acid
lucidin	magnesium	methyl oleate	morindadiol
morindanigrine	morindin	morindone	myristic acid
nonanoic acid	nordamnacanthal	octanoic acid	oleic acid
palmitic acid	parrafin	pectins	pentose
phosphate	physcion	potassium	protein
resins	rhamnose	ricinoleic acid	rubiadin
scopoletin	sitosterol	sodium	B-sitosterol
stearic acid	sterols	stigmasterol	terpenoids
ursolic acid	vitamin C	vomifoliol	wax

intrinsic components of noni, it can lower blood pressure to unhealthy levels. On the other hand, when scopoletin is ingested in whole food form, it does not have this effect. Experts have theorized that this phenomenon is the result of a combined effect from a number of noni components acting together to regulate blood pressure in a synergistic way. In other words, mother nature knows what she's doing.

HOW DOES NONI WORK? A CLOSER LOOK AT THEORIES ON MORINDA CITRIFOLIA

Formal scientific research on noni may be just a dozen or so years in the making, but we have already uncovered numerous clues into the exact mechanisms that give noni its healing properties. Discoveries about how noni works are still in preliminary stages, but the evidence that has surfaced so far is worth getting excited about. I have already mentioned some of the studies that have been published about noni and introduced you to some of noni's more promising compounds. Now, let me briefly introduce you to some of the emerging theories that explain how noni works.

A Crash Course in Adaptogens

As mentioned earlier, a one-size-fits-all approach to multiple ailments often results in skepticism from the medical community. Once again, it must be stressed that noni contains a broad range of compounds that work on a cellular level. Furthermore, many of noni's properties, like its pain killing ability, have multiple uses. The fact that noni can either lower or raise blood pressure attests to its true adaptogenic nature. It's role as an adaptogenic herb is very important to complementary and alternative medicine and worth further discussion.

Our health (and our survival) depends on our ability to adapt to our environment. Chronic stress—caused by a failure to adapt—has been linked to diseases like irritable bowel, heart disease, PMS, obesity, fibromyalgia, depression and even cancer. Overexposure to stress hormones can compromise our immune systems and leave us vulnerable to a multitude of illnesses. Adaptogenic plants like noni affect the immune, endocrine and nervous system, and by strengthening those systems, increase the body's capability to adapt to both internal and external stressors. Many plants are known to counteract the negative effects of stress. One of the most well-known adaptogens is ginseng, which is used to treat a number of health problems. Reishi mushroom is another. In fact, adaptogenic plants have been used in Chinese medicine for thousands of years.

A plant is considered adaptogenic if it has a "non-specific action" in the body. In other words, it helps the body adapt to a variety of internal and external stresses without the harmful side effects seen with synthetic drugs. Adaptogens often work by helping the body make better use of energy supplies or by helping it repair damaged cells and tissues and improve vital functions. Noni's adaptogenic effects will become more clear in the following section.

Heinicke's "Xeronine System"

Knowledge about xeronine is imperative to understanding how noni functions. Dr. Ralph Heinicke, if you remember, is a leader in noni research, and he has developed a theory that places xeronine as the compound behind noni's therapeutic actions. Heinicke's research began in the 1950s while he was studying a compound in pineapple called *bromelain*. At the time, bromelain was being used to treat chronic pain, arthritis and even cancer, and this sparked the interest of numerous pharmaceutical companies. Interestingly, purified bromelain testing conducted by drug companies yielded few positive results, which perplexed Heinicke and his colleagues. After researching the medicinal uses for bromelain extracts, however, Heinicke isolated a substance called proxeronine, which promotes the production of xeronine in the body (when combined with the enzyme proxeroninase and other compounds). Xeronine, as discussed earlier in the chapter, aids in normal cell function and proxeronine is needed for the body to produce xeronine.

Because xeronine affects the health of the body at the cellular level, it influences the function of every body system.

Heinicke decided that proxeronine must be the key to brome-lain's effectiveness. The purified bromelain that was tested by the FDA contained no proxeronine because it was all removed during the purification process.

Eventually, Heinicke realized that although pineapple is a good source of proxeronine, noni was an even better source. It is, in fact, the best known source of proxeronine and is many times stronger than pineapple. Furthermore, proxero-nine is found in limited supply in the body.

Research into xeronine has determined that the brain directs the release of proxeronine from the liver into the bloodstream every few hours so that tissues and organs can take the proxeronine they need to produce xeronine for cell maintenance and repair. However, there is only enough prox-eronine in the body for normal cell repair in healthy individ-uals. But a body under stress has insufficient proxeronine supplies to repair cells. This means when the body is taxed by the presence of cancerous cells, a chronic infection or danger-ous levels of environmental toxins, it may not have enough proxeronine to fix itself.

To test his theory he gave a xeronine solution isolated from noni to mice infected with a deadly toxin called *tetrodotoxin*. Those mice who were not treated with xeronine died. However, those mice given xeronine not only lived, they also showed no symptoms of infection. Even after repeated test-ing, the results were the same. Similar testing and anecdotal research seem to support these findings.

The Nitric Oxide Connection

Although the last chapter provided an introduction to nitric oxide, noni's link to this amazing substance deserves further discussion, especially when discussing how noni works. You may have heard about some of the research on nitric oxide and blood pressure; in fact, as mentioned earlier, scientists studying nitric oxide were awarded the Nobel prize

"My life was changed forever"

"My life was changed forever in December of 1998. That was when I was first introduced to noni juice.

My friend Rhonda had been telling my husband about noni juice for some time as she felt it would help our son Mitchell with a very severe asthma condition. I was very skeptical and almost let my negative feelings about life at that time stop me from even trying the juice.

Before I would give it to Mitchell, I wanted to try it first. At that time I was suffering from an eye infection, severe allergies and asthma. That night, with my first ounce of noni juice, I had the best sleep I had in years! When I woke up, I couldn't believe that I didn't need my asthma medicine even once . . . I began taking 2 ounces per day and have noticed many benefits such as more energy, no more back or leg pain, a feeling of positive well-being and my asthma and allergies seldom, if ever, bother me.

With benefits like this, I obviously wanted to share this with my entire family. My husband and four children . . . have all received various benefits. The most dramatic is my son Mitchell. His biggest health challenge, asthma, almost cost him his life twice. Noni juice is the only natural health supplement that has been able to get him off steroids. We are confident that with continued use of noni juice, the long term side effects from prolonged steroid use can be reversed.

We have all heard the saying "If you have your health you have everything." You don't know how true that is until you lose it! My family and I will continue to drink noni juice every day. It is a big part of our lives."

Valerie A., Canada

for medicine in 1998. Discovered in the eighties, nitric oxide (*Science* magazine's recent "Molecule of the Year") has been the subject of hundreds of studies. It relaxes and expands blood vessel walls, making it useful for not only high blood pressure, but also a number of cardiovascular conditions. In fact, research seems to show that nitric oxide is essential for the normal functioning of almost every system of the body. Moreover, it affects immunity, brain function, intestinal activity, airway and heart function, and body movement.

Many specific properties of nitric oxide have already been identified and studied. For example, its ability to relax arteries and artery walls make it useful for treating high blood pressure and angina, and it also may lower LDL (bad) cholesterol by scavenging free radicals and prevent blood clots that cause strokes. Its effect on insulin secretion make it useful for preventing or treating diabetes, and it also influences the release of human growth hormone (HGH) and the effectiveness of certain immune cells. Its effects on the brain and nervous system have also been studied, and it has been found to increase blood flow to brain cells and enhances long-term memory. It also makes communication between the brain and nerve cells more effective, and it has been used to treat impotence and certain types of cancer.

Although noni does not contain nitric oxide, it appears to promote its biosynthesis. Published studies from Hawaii have found that the body's production of nitric oxide can be stimulated by ingesting noni. In fact, one 1997 study found that noni supplementation boosted macrophage (immune cell) activity, which was attributed to higher levels of nitric oxide in the body. Noni's effects on nitric oxide production might explain noni's usefulness in treating microbial infections, cardiovascular problems and cancer.

Now that you have a good idea about how noni works and are familiar with the most important noni components, let's see how these compounds can be used to improve various health conditions, not to mention overall health.

CHAPTER FOUR

Noni for Increased Energy

- What is chronic fatigue?
- Symptoms of fatigue
- How can noni help boost energy levels?

- Using noni for fibromyalgia and CFS
- Other ways to fight fatigue

All of us have felt fatigued at some time or another in our lives—after skipping a meal, not getting enough sleep or finishing an intense exercise session. Colds, flu and other infections are often accompanied by fatigue. But what happens when our energy levels are low every week or every day?

If you find yourself feeling fatigued more often than usual, you are not alone. More and more Americans are having trouble sleeping and are waking unrefreshed. In addition, many are so tired during the day that their ability to concentrate and execute tasks is significantly impaired. Many suffer from "whole-body fatigue" that is not relieved by sleep. In fact, a 2000 study by the National Sleep Foundation found nearly half of adults surveyed were severely fatigued a few days or more per month and that it interfered with daily activities. And one in five surveyed said they felt this fatigue at least three days a week.

The rise in the number of people with a chronic lack of energy is not surprising. Most Americans are getting less than seven hours of sleep a night during the work week and some even less. Many are victims of chronic stress because of overwhelming demands from family and the workplace. Combining a fast-paced life with poor eating habits, a lack of exercise and poor sleep makes for a disastrous health combination. Moreover, fatigue may originate from specific health problems like chronic fatigue syndrome, fibromyalgia or even cancer. Even a low-grade sinus infection will sap energy if it is not treated. Sometimes the cause of persistent fatigue remains a mystery, but some possible causes of fatigue are listed in the accompanying side bar.

WHAT IS CHRONIC FATIGUE?

Persistent fatigue is not the occasional tiredness we all experience from time to time, but rather an ongoing, generalized lack of energy that affects the entire body and is not relieved by sleep. Acute fatigue is defined as having symptoms

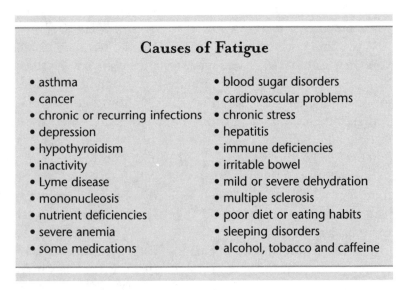

Causes of Fatigue

- asthma
- cancer
- chronic or recurring infections
- depression
- hypothyroidism
- inactivity
- Lyme disease
- mononucleosis
- nutrient deficiencies
- severe anemia
- some medications
- blood sugar disorders
- cardiovascular problems
- chronic stress
- hepatitis
- immune deficiencies
- irritable bowel
- mild or severe dehydration
- multiple sclerosis
- poor diet or eating habits
- sleeping disorders
- alcohol, tobacco and caffeine

for one month, and if you have chronic fatigue, you have had symptoms for at least six months. Fatigue can mean sleepiness, lack of stamina, muscle weakness or a combination of these symptoms. You may have one bout of fatigue and then be fine, or you could have a cycle of chronic fatigue, where you have periods of normal energy followed by periods of profound fatigue.

No one really knows what triggers recurring cycles of chronic fatigue, but some speculate that periods of physical or emotional stress may be to blame. The most damaging side effect of persistent fatigue is its interference in a person's ability to function and their quality of life. Fatigue is particularly debilitating for those with immune deficiencies, fibromyalgia, chronic fatigue syndrome (CFS) and cancer (especially cancer patients undergoing chemotherapy and/or radiation therapy).

SYMPTOMS OF CHRONIC FATIGUE

- depression
- tired eyes
- decreased concentration
- irritability
- whole-body weakness
- achy muscles
- stiff shoulders
- decreased energy
- general malaise
- lack of motivation
- sleepiness
- anxiety
- nervousness
- sleeping disturbances

HOW CAN NONI HELP BOOST ENERGY LEVELS?

Whether you suffer from occasional or persistent fatigue, you may benefit from taking noni. In the previous chapter, we referred to noni as an adaptogenic plant, meaning that it can help the body adapt to changes in the environment, both the physical and the psychological stressors. If you recall, one of the ways that adaptogens work is by helping the body make better use of energy. Anecdotal evidence supports noni's ability to boost energy levels, and although scientific studies on noni have not supplied us with all the answers, they point to noni's impact on energy use and conservation in the body. Let's quickly review how the body makes energy.

The Krebs Cycle

How does the body create the energy it needs to function? Simply stated, our bodies get their energy from food, but the actual process of creating energy is a bit more complicated. I won't delve into the nitty gritty of energy production, but let's review a few basic ideas so we can better understand what noni may contribute to the process.

The Krebs cycle is simply the process by which the body produces energy. Each cell contains structures called *mitochondria*, which are responsible for converting substances like vitamins, minerals and proteins into energy that can be used by the body (called adenosine triphosphate or ATP). Without ATP, the body would not be able to execute even the most basic functions.

If anything interferes with the production of energy by the body, such as cell malfunction or an inability to obtain all of the necessary substances and enzymes to produce ATP energy, then the health of the body suffers. In fact, even a relatively minor flaw in generating energy can create a serious problem.

If the body is not producing the energy it needs to function at optimal levels, some of the body's needs will not be met. Consequently, an individual's overall health will suffer. Basically, symptoms of fatigue are just the body's way of letting you know that its energy needs are not being met.

Of course, the reasons why certain people are inefficient in their energy production are not always clear. Scientists do not yet have all the answers, but it is clear that immune function, illness and stress all play a role.

What Can Noni Do?

Although the exact mechanisms which allow noni to affect energy production are unknown, we do know that noni affects health on the cellular level. Noni stimulates the body to produce xeronine and nitric oxide. Both of these substances have broad-ranging effects on the health of the body because they promote the health of cells. In fact, noni may directly influence cell mitochondria and other vital parts of cells. We also know that energy required by the body to function is delivered by and produced in cells. Noni's adaptogenic qualities help the body use energy more efficiently—a fact supported by anecdotal evidence and historical usage. In fact, noni has been used by mountain climbers and marathoners because of its energy-boosting properties. Furthermore, research on noni has shown that it positively affects the immune system. If your fatigue is the result of an ongoing infection or major illness, noni may give your body the extra boost it needs to recover.

We are learning that some people harbor hidden viral, bacterial or parasitic infections that can go untreated for years, causing unexplained fatigue and even depression. If your immune system must deal with a chronic infection, it saps strength from the rest of the body. One example is an ongoing tooth or gum infection that places an enormous strain on the body's defenses and may even contribute to ailments in seemingly unrelated body systems. By supplying the body with an immune booster, these infections may be resolved and the health of all of your body systems can improve. Noni's immune boosting properties will be discussed in more detail in the next chapter.

USING NONI FOR FIBROMYALGIA AND CFS

Noni may be useful for those suffering with fibromyalgia and chronic fatigue syndrome because of its energy-boosting effects. Both syndromes are characterized by depression, sleep disorders and ever-present fatigue, as well as other symptoms. Fibromyalgics also suffer from chronic pain in specific places called "tender points." The medical community still knows relatively little about what causes these syndromes or how to treat and/or reverse them. Yet millions of Americans are currently diagnosed with fibromyalgia or CFS.

Traditional treatments usually include antidepressants, sleeping pills and pain medication (for fibromyalgia). However, noni may offer new hope to suffers of CFS and fibromyalgia because of its powerful effects on energy levels, pain and the immune system. Research on damnacanthal in noni fruit found it was able to inhibit the Epstein-Barr virus. There are established links between this virus and diseases like chronic fatigue syndrome. Many scientists believe that weakened immune systems may be to blame for these syndromes, and noni's immune-boosting properties may prove helpful against these weaknesses. Furthermore, the ability of noni to normalize cell function may also be helpful for those with CFS and fibromyalgia. Some experts theorize that neurotransmitter abnormalities may be at the root of these syndromes. Noni's normalizing effects on cells may be able to repair these abnormalities.

Anecdotal evidence supports using noni for CFS and fibromyalgia. Noni's effects on these syndromes were even more profound when individuals combined noni supplementation with proper diet, regular exercise, a multi-vitamin/mineral supplement and mind-body therapies like meditation.

OTHER WAYS TO FIGHT FATIGUE

Exercise. Start moving! Although exercise may seem like the last thing you want to do when you are chronically fatigued, its benefits are beyond measure—especially aerobic exercise. The word *aerobic* means "air life" in Greek, a definition that could not be more appropriate. Aerobic doesn't refer to cardiovascular exercise alone. It also describes how the body produces energy and stays alive. Aerobic metabolism is the phrase referring to the body's use of oxygen to make energy, and as you know, the body cannot survive without oxygen. Walking, running, biking and swimming all give the body a cardiovascular workout and are therefore considered aerobic. In addition to aerobic exercise, you should also start a strength training and flexibility program. Of course, consult with a physician before beginning any exercise program.

Exercise increases blood flow to the muscles, boosts the body's supply of feel-good endorphins and serotonin, and enhances T-cell (an immune cell) and growth hormone production. Research shows that regular exercisers also sleep better, are less anxious and depressed, and are less likely to suffer with heart and blood sugar problems. The value of regular exercise for women of all ages cannot be overly emphasized, and women are more at risk for developing chronic fatigue. I've heard women profess on more than one occasion that exercising has preserved their well-being and saved their sanity. Exercising can minimize the hormonally induced miseries that characterize menopause and ease menstrual cramps, as well as the stress created by the ebb and flow of hormones.

The key successful to exercising is to start slowly and grad-

"Noni has given me fantastic energy!"

"I was an overworked, stressed out journalist working sixty hours a week. After thirty-seven years in the media, I am now an evangelist for noni juice. When a friend handed me a bottle about two years ago and told me I might get a benefit, I really didn't believe him. How could a funny juice from the islands help me? Well, after only six weeks on the juice, I was a new man. (It didn't impress my girlfriend though, because she didn't want a new man—she was happy with me.)

But seriously, noni juice has given me fantastic energy, my sleep patterns are better, and the back pain I had for ten years is gone. I now travel the world telling people about noni juice, and I will take it until the day I die. Although, now that I am on the juice that could be a long way off!"

Paul M., Australia

ually build from where you started. Keep your routine practical and simple. Choose the time of day that gives you the best chance for success. Use music to enhance your exercise routine. Music works to motivate and energize your body so you move faster for longer periods of time.

What are the three best exercises? Walking, walking and more walking. Walk around the block after work, walk a dog, walk where and when it's safe, and walk every day. Brisk walking is especially good and if you walk rapidly for even ten minutes a day, you can expect to feel a considerable mental lift and energy surge. Always keep in mind that some exercise (no matter how small) is infinitely better than none. Keep your goals realistic or you'll stop altogether. Ideally, you should (at least) be walking for thirty minutes three to five times a week at a brisk pace and doing weight-bearing exercises and strength training for at least thirty minutes three times a week. Increasing your cardio workout to forty-five or more minutes a session is even better.

Diet. Keep your blood sugar stable by eating smaller meals more frequently. Do not go longer than four hours without eating. Eating three small meals and two healthy snacks each day is a great option. Eat a variety of whole grains and vegetables. Take a multivitamin and mineral supplement daily.

Stay away from "high glycemic" foods. In other words, reduce your intake of simple carbohydrates like white bread and sugar, which are converted into glucose quickly by the body and can cause extreme blood sugar fluctuations. Meals containing complex carbohydrates and healthy protein will help keep blood sugar in normal ranges. Soy, whole grains, nuts and seeds are great choices. Pick foods high in fiber and potassium. Be careful not to skimp on complex carbohydrates as some fad diets recommend. Low-carbohydrate diets can cause fatigue and depression, and they have been linked to other serious health problems.

For higher energy levels, cut out caffeine and alcohol and stay hydrated. Many Americans are mildly dehydrated and don't even know it. Symptoms of dehydration include fatigue and headaches. Drink sixty-four ounces of water a day, and remember that caffeine is a diuretic, so you will need to consume an extra eight ounces of water for every can of soda or cup of coffee.

Sleep. Undoubtedly, sleep disturbances can both cause chronic fatigue and depression, or can result from its presence. Some scientists believe that the wrong kind of sleep initiates depression and chronic fatigue. They suggest that the chemical changes which occur in the brain during sleep may have a direct bearing on the nerves and neurotransmitters that produce mood and a sense of well-being. Perhaps this finally explains the existence of "morning people." We need to get adequate amounts of REM (rapid eye movement) sleep for an extended period of time or serious health consequences can result. REM sleep is the stage of sleep when we dream and do a great deal of cellular repair and regeneration. If you lack REM sleep, protein production in the brain is inhibited, and cellular repair is compromised in virtually every body system.

Be aware also that a continual lack of quality sleep can actually accumulate over time. This sleep debt can result in subtle, unexplained symptoms. In addition, if you take any kind of drug, you may be significantly compromising the quality of your sleep. Sedatives, stimulants like caffeine, anticonvulsants and antihistamines are just a few of the many chemical agents that interfere with normal sleep patterns, causing daytime fatigue. Sleep apnea, or abnormal breathing, can deprive brain cells of adequate oxygen. A repeated lack of oxygen to brain tissue can result in mental fogginess, fatigue and forgetfulness. In addition, food allergies are notorious for causing insomnia or restless sleep, especially in children.

To reduce sleep-related fatigue, establish a regular schedule for when you go to bed and get up in the morning (even on weekends). Get regular exercise and begin a bedtime routine to relax you so you can more easily fall asleep. Read a book, take a bath or do a fifteen-minute meditation with some yoga—whatever unwinds you. Avoid eating large meals after seven or eight in the evening. Also, try to keep the atmosphere in the bedroom as soothing as possible—dark, cool and with a comfortable bed. Try not to read or eat in bed. Keep the bed as a place where you go to sleep. If you need a noise to lull you to sleep, purchase a white noise machine or use sound boxes (ocean tides, rainfall, falling water, crickets, etc.).

Relax. If you are overwhelmed with responsibilities, consider delegating or overhauling your schedule. You may even decide to switch jobs. Do daily meditation or yoga. If you are not the "yoga" type, try simple stretching and breathing exercises. Many experts also recommend daily journal writing or taking a stress management course. Do whatever it takes to develop better coping skills. The negative effects of chronic stress are severe and should not be ignored.

Complementary herbs: ginseng, kelp, spirulina, bee pollen, suma, gotu kola

If you use noni and some of the above methods to fight fatigue, you are bound to notice a number of other health benefits that accompany your increased energy. You will probably sleep better, become more active and suffer fewer illnesses and bouts of depression. In fact, noni's abilities to increase energy and boost the immune system go hand in hand. Let's look at how noni affects your ability to fight off illness in more detail.

CHAPTER FIVE

Noni and the Immune System

- Immune system basics
- Immune system disorders
- Mainstream medicine and the immune system
- Prevention is the best medicine
- Noni: powerful immune booster
- Noni for microbe infections
- HIV and noni
- Treating allergies with noni
- Other ways to boost immunity

In the last chapter, I listed immune system dysfunction as a cause for chronic low energy. A weakened or compromised immune system can manifest itself in many other ways. If you suffer from chronic colds or sinus infections or if it seems like you get every virus that goes around the office, your immunity could use a good boost. Chronic illnesses, even seemingly minor problems like a low-grade ear infection or seasonal allergies, tax immune cells over time and drain you of needed energy. Ultimately, the combined effect of these small ailments on your immune system may be far greater than you imagine—even determining your cancer risk, how you recover from major injuries or surgeries, and even how you age.

Why? If too many demands are made on your body (and your immune system) and your diet or lifestyle does not meet those needs, disease will result. This deficit could manifest itself as chronic fatigue, infections, migraines and other pain, hormone imbalances, depression, or if it is severe, by the appearance of serious diseases like fibromyalgia or cancer. If you suffer from health problems like these, your body could be trying to tell you that it doesn't have sufficient resources to provide you with optimal health protection. It has to cut corners, which leaves you more vulnerable to major and minor illnesses.

The negative effects of chronic stress and poor health on the body—and specifically the immune system—can be immense. Lack of sleep, inactivity and poor diet all contribute to a weakened immune system because each denies the body of essential components that it needs to function properly. Environmental hazards like pollution and toxins can also deplete your immune system's resources. And if these resources are spread too thin, you become vulnerable. For example, if you suffer regularly from sinus infections, your immune system is diverting valuable energy to this preventable problem that it could be using to fight off more dangerous threats, like cancer.

The key to being healthy and living long is a strong immune system. Why treat an existing illness when you may be able to prevent it altogether? It is easier (and less expensive) to prevent diseases (large or small) than trying to treat them after the fact. And if you are injured or need surgery, a strong immune system increases your chances of survival and a speedy recovery.

I have already spoken about the importance of eating right and exercising for overall health, but for most of us, this is not enough. But by taking nutritional supplements, we give ourselves the extra protection we need to fight off diseases and other threats. Noni is a wonderful option because it offers a variety of benefits, including proven benefits for the immune system. Let's take a minute to review what the immune system is, how it works and what happens when the immune system malfunctions.

IMMUNE SYSTEM BASICS

The immune system is a highly complex network of cells and organs located throughout the body that defend it against attacks by foreign invaders like bacteria, fungi, parasites and viruses. It also helps rid the body of other foreign substances and malignant cells. Among these immune organs are the tonsils, the thymus, spleen, appendix, lymph nodes and bone marrow. They are called "lymphoid organs" because they are in charge of the growth, development and use of white blood cells called *lymphocytes*, which are essential to immune function. Although these organs are located in different points in the body, they function together through the lymphatic system, a network of vessels (similar to blood vessels) where immune and foreign cells are channeled in clear fluid called *lymph*. To facilitate this process, small structures called *lymph nodes* are located at various check points where immune cells can collect and confront antigens (foreign cells and particles).

How Do Immune Cells Recognize Invaders?

The basic duties of the immune system are to identify invaders, distinguish them from the body's own cells and rid the body of any threats. Every cell in the body carries molecules called *self markers* that identify it as belonging to the body, and under normal conditions the body's immune cells do not attack cells with these markers.

Foreign bodies also have distinctive markers. Amazingly, the immune system not only recognizes and distinguishes among millions of different foreign molecules, but it also responds to and counteracts them individually by producing immune cells called *antibodies*. Antibodies are triggered by the presence of any foreign substance (called an *antigen*). Bacteria are antigens, as are cells from someone else (which is why a transplanted organ can be rejected by the body).

A Closer Look at Immune Cells

Immune cells originate in stem cells located in the bone marrow. There are various types of immune cells, but they can be divided into a few main groups. For instance, large white blood cells that devour cells and particles are called *phagocytes* (and include cells such as macrophages and monocytes) and are collectively known as *myeloid cells*. Phagocytes are just one type of myeloid cell. B and T cells are classes of small white blood cells called lymphocytes.

B cells are very important because they secrete antibodies, immune cells that belong to a family of protein molecules known as *immunoglobulins* (of which there are nine identified classes, among them IgG, IgA, IgM, IgE and IgD, each with their own duties). In fact, each B cell makes one specific antibody designed to react to one type of antigen. When a B cell is triggered by an antigen, large plasma cells respond and manufacture the necessary antibody. Each antibody has unique contours on one side that allow it to bind to its matching antigen. The antibody fits the antigen perfectly—like a key fits into a lock. The other side of the antibody is able to link to other immune cells.

Some immunoglobulins—such as IgG—may sound more familiar than others. There are four types of IgG immunoglobulins, and they are found in the blood. IgA guards body entrances and is found in tears and saliva. Others are found only in trace amounts, like IgE; however, if you suffer from allergies, IgE is responsible for those itchy, sneezy symptoms.

T cells, probably one of the most well known immune cells, provide a dual immune defense—helping to regulate immune function and destroy foreign cells. Regulatory T cells activate or suppress other immune cells, while cytotoxic T cells are responsible for disposing of infected and cancerous cells. These cells are also the ones that trigger the body to reject organs and tissue transplants.

Cytotoxic T cells are one type of immune killer cell; other type is natural killer (NK) cells. Whereas cytotoxic T cells need to identify a particular antigen in order to attack, NK cells do not. Both types are potent destroyers, however, and kill on contact.

Another group of cells you may have heard of is the cytokines. Cytokines are messengers that recruit other cells in the event of an invader attack. They do this by attaching to certain sites on the cells. Once attached, they can encourage cell growth, activation and movement, or they can destroy targeted cells. One example of a cell targeted by cytokines would be a cancerous cell, which is a normal cell that has mutated. Cytokines are also called *interleukins* because they can send messages between white blood cells (leukocytes).

As mentioned earlier, phagocytes are large white blood cells that devour cells and particles, including monocytes (in blood), macrophages (in tissue) and neutrophils (in blood and tissue). Macrophages are probably the best known of these scavengers and also activate T cells.

In addition to these immune cells are circulating proteins, part of a complementary system that help antibodies destroy invaders. These proteins are found in the blood and are activated when they encounter an antibody attached to a foreign invader. Each complement protein has its own job to perform in order to break through the protective membrane of the targeted cell so that it may be destroyed.

Immune Defense: Running the Gauntlet

But how do microbes and other invaders get into the body in the first place? Microbes must survive a number of barriers, the first of which is the skin and accompanying mucous membranes that not only physically impede the progress of invaders but also contain scavenger cells and antibodies. If the invader cells make it past these barriers, they are greeted with patrolling scavenger cells, complement proteins and various other defenses that attack anything that they determine is not supposed to be there. These defenses are nonspecific, meaning that they are not targeted toward any specific invader, but to foreign cells in general.

Foreign agents tough enough to survive these defenses are then greeted by weapons (antibodies and other immune cells) specifically targeted for them (hopefully). In fact, almost every antigen triggers specific and nonspecific defense responses by the body. Cells are able to recognize their targets because of customized molecules called *antigen receptors* that they carry, which can function in simple or very sophisticated ways to identify and destroy threats.

Memory: The Key to Immunity

With so many foreign threats, how does the body keep track of all possible antigens? Moreover, how can it possibly defend against so many? Well, the immune system has developed ways to remember the invaders it encounters. Whenever T cells and B cells respond to a threat, some of them become memory cells, so that the next time the same invader shows up again, the immune system will recall how it originally defended itself. If there are long-term memory cells for an antigen, it can be destroyed very quickly. Vaccines work on this premise: by exposing the body to inactive or very small amounts of an infectious microbe, vaccines can trigger the creation of memory cells. By doing so, if the body is exposed to the "real thing," it can fight off the threat without incident.

The immune system also has a "short-term memory," meaning that it can receive antibodies from another individual and use the memory of these antibodies to fight off an invader. A great example of this is the antibody protection a fetus receives from its mother.

IMMUNE SYSTEM DISORDERS

Because the immune system is so complex and so many things can interfere with its duties, it doesn't always function properly. When this happens, the body loses the protection it needs to fight off disease and illness. Immune dysfunction can be aggravated by illness and poor health habits. Let's look at some examples of faulty immunity.

Allergies. As mentioned earlier, allergies are linked to the IgE antibody. Although usually found only in trace amounts in the body, a person with an allergy will have much higher amounts of this antibody. For instance, the immune cells of a person with a sensitivity to a particular pollen will produce large amounts of an IgE antibody at their first exposure. These IgE antibodies attach to cells in the lungs, skin, tongue, nose and gastrointestinal tract called mast cells, so the next time the person is exposed to the allergen, these mast cells release large amounts of chemicals that cause sneezing, hives and other symptoms.

Autoimmune diseases. At the beginning of this section, I mentioned that immune cells are geared to attack cells that they do not recognize as their own. However, if the immune system's ability to recognize cells deteriorates, the body begins to attack its own cells or organs by producing antibodies (called autoantibodies) and T cells that are directed at the body's own cells. Autoantibodies are at the root of many diseases. For example, diabetics may have T cells that attack the body's pancreas, and rheumatic individuals may produce autoantibodies that cause arthritic symptoms.

HIV/AIDS. AIDS is an example of an immunodeficiency disorder. This disease is caused when the immune system loses at least one of its components, either through an inherited condition or because of something acquired (like HIV). Immunodeficiencies can also be a side effect of drugs or other treatments—such as seen in cancer patients undergoing chemotherapy. AIDS is caused by a virus that destroys T cells (specifically helper T cells). In fact, the immunity-destroying virus is harbored in the immune system's own macrophages and T cells. The virus is spread from cell to cell by mutations of the cell's DNA (the cell's genetic material).

Cancer. Cancerous cells are produced by the body every day, but they are usually eliminated by patrolling immune cells designed to search the entire body each day and remove mutated (malignant) cells. When a cell becomes cancerous, it loses its self marker, signifying to the body's immune defenses that it needs to be disposed of. When this process of identifying and eliminating rogue cells fails, tumors develop. Theories as to why this process fails are plentiful, but some experts feel that at least one explanation is that this failure is the result of a weakened or overwhelmed immune system. We will discuss cancer in more detail in the next chapter.

MAINSTREAM MEDICINE AND THE IMMUNE SYSTEM

No one can deny the importance of vaccines and antibiotics in reducing deaths caused by serious illness or disease; however, scientists are now beginning to see how our dependence on these treatments can backfire. The emergence of drug-resistant bacteria is largely the result of antibiotic overprescription and misuse. In fact, many prescriptions and medical treatments can ultimately (directly or indirectly) weaken the immune system and actually leave us more vulnerable to future illness or secondary infections. Cancer treatments are notorious for this, along with many other conventional methods for fighting illness. These therapies often cripple the immune system by short circuiting the body's natural defenses. This sometimes adversarial relationship between medicine and immunity may often leave the body more vulnerable. Instead of enhancing the immune system, some medical treatments circumvent or suppress natural immune function. Over time, this results in an immune system that is not equipped to handle threats without assistance.

In addition, as mentioned in **Chapter 1**, modern medicine tends to focus on treating the symptoms of disease rather than the causes (or better yet, preventing disease altogether). Because of this focus, the immune system may be more easily overworked and overwhelmed. How? Masking the symptoms of a problem may make it more bearable, but it does not relieve the burden placed on your immune system. Repeated and chronic illnesses, even small ones, put added stress on your immune system as well.

PREVENTION IS THE BEST MEDICINE

Clearly the best strategy for immune strength is to prevent illness whenever possible. Ideally, we should eradicate existing health problems by focusing on the causes of disease rather than alleviating symptoms. One strength of complementary and alternative medicine is its emphasis on cause and prevention. CAM treatments work with your immune system—not in spite of it. A great example is the common natural cold-and-flu treatment called echinacea. Research on echinacea has found that it stimulates the immune system by increasing the number of leukocytes (white blood cells) and splenocytes (white blood cells in the spleen) while enhancing phagocyte (large white blood cells) and granulocyte (granular white blood cells) activity. It fights bacteria by working with your body's own defenses. Antibiotics, on the other hand, work by killing bacteria or preventing the growth of bacteria. They offer no immune boost whatsoever, killing good bacteria along with the bad. To an antibiotic, all bacteria are created equal.

NONI: POWERFUL IMMUNE BOOSTER

Noni is like echinacea in that it works with the immune system to fight and prevent illness. Earlier I mentioned that noni is an adaptogenic herb. Overexposure to stress hormones compromises our immune systems leaving us vulnerable to illness and disease. Adaptogenic plants like noni affect our immune, endocrine and nervous systems, increasing our ability to adapt to internal and external stress.

A 1999 study in *Phytotherapy* found that noni fruit contains polysaccharides that enhance immune function. There is evidence, for instance, that noni may help increase T-cell counts. T cells are especially important to the immune system because they provide a dual immune defense—regulating immune function and destroying foreign cells. In fact, noni's antitumor properties have been attributed in part to its ability to stimulate T-cell production.

Moreover, noni alkaloids have the ability to boost phagocytosis, a process where white blood cells called *phagocytes* attack and consume foreign cells. Noni also enhances macrophage and lymphocyte activity and regulates thymocytes. The University of Hawaii has also identified other immune cells that are enhanced by noni, including interleukins 1, 2, 4, 10 and 12; interferon and lipopolysaccharide.

A 1999 study found that ursolic acid in the noni leaf positively impacts the immune system as well, which may not only help prevent cancer, but also fight off various viral, bacterial and fungal infections. Noni also contains vitamin C, an excellent immune booster.

Some experts theorize that the proxeronine in noni (which stimulates xeronine production in the body) may also positively affect immunity. Xeronine, if you remember, is a compound involved in healthy cell regulation. It helps maintain healthy cells and encourages abnormal cells to regain normal function. Since it works on a cellular level, it may beneficially affect every body system, including the immune system.

Noni also prompts the body to produce nitric oxide. Research has shown that nitric oxide is essential for the normal functioning of almost every system of the body, including the immune system. It affects the release of human growth hormone (HGH) and the effectiveness of certain immune cells. In fact, nitric oxide has been used to treat certain types of cancer. We will discuss noni's cancer applications in more detail in the next chapter.

NONI FOR MICROBE INFECTIONS

Bioactive components in the whole noni plant have a demonstrated ability to fight several different microbes, including bacteria, viruses and fungi. Noni has proven effects against several types of bacteria including: *Escherichia coli*, *Salmonella typhosa* (and other types), *Shigella paradysenteriae*, *M. pyrogenes*, *Pseudomonas aeruginosa*, *Proteus morganii*, *Bacillus subtilis* and *Staphylococcus aureus*. Noni's antimicrobial properties may explain why it is used to treat colds and flu.

In addition, damnacanthal, a substance found in noni, has been shown to inhibit Epstein-Barr virus in its early stages. Epstein-Barr often occurs in people with weak immune systems and is linked to chronic fatigue syndrome. And in the Philippines, noni is used to rid the body of parasites, disinfect wounds, and heal stomach ulcers (often caused by bacteria). Other studies suggest that the scopoletin in noni may inhibit the actions of the dangerous *E. coli* bacteria. Noni's antimicrobial power makes it an excellent supplement for treating earaches, acne, eye infections, intestinal parasites, ringworm, sore throat, gum disease, and urinary tract, sinus and other infections.

HIV AND NONI

As mentioned earlier in the chapter, AIDS is an example of an immunodeficiency disorder caused by a virus (HIV or human immunodeficiency virus) which destroys helper T cells. The virus is harbored in the immune system's own macrophages and T cells and is spread from cell to cell by DNA mutations. A person is diagnosed as having AIDS when their T cell count falls below 200 (a normal T cell count is 600–1,000), or they have developed a serious infection (called an "opportunistic infection") that they would not have contracted if the virus wasn't present. There is more than one type of HIV, but all eventually cause AIDS, and the symptoms accompanying the disease vary greatly. Common symptoms include recurring infections, swollen lymph glands, night sweating and fever, coughing, skin lesions, white spots in the mouth, irritable bowel, weight loss and pneumonia. Secondary infections like yeast and respiratory infections are especially dangerous for those with HIV or full-blown AIDS because of their weakened immune systems.

Noni offers hope both for treating the virus that causes AIDS and secondary or opportunistic infections that result from having the virus. In fact, noni has appeared as a viable treatment in the medical journal *AIDS Patient Care Studies* as recently as 2001. Noni treatment for HIV and AIDS is beneficial because of the immune enhancing power of the plant. Noni is believed to not only boost T cell counts but also stimulate the activity and production of various immune cells. In addition, because noni prompts the production of xeronine, it can potentially repair cells damaged by the HIV virus.

Although research in this area still needs to be done, anecdotal evidence suggests that noni may offer individuals with HIV another way to boost immune function while taking conventional antiviral medications for the disease. Of course, before using noni for any serious condition, it is important to discuss possible contraindications with your doctor.

TREATING ALLERGIES WITH NONI

Allergies are the result of an immune dysfunction where the body responds to a potential allergen by producing too much IgE. These IgE antibodies attach to cells in the lungs, skin, tongue, nose and gastrointestinal tract, so the next time the person is exposed, the body responds by sneezing and/or producing hives (and other symptoms). Using noni for allergies is another area largely unexplored by traditional medical research. Based on noni's effects on malfunctioning cells and on the immune system, it is probable that noni may relieve allergies in some people. In fact, many individuals who have experienced relief from allergies have attributed their success to noni.

OTHER WAYS TO BOOST IMMUNITY

Nutritional Supplements. Various vitamins and minerals can boost immune function. Vitamins A, D and C, iron, manganese and zinc are all necessary for optimal immune function. Flavonoids, DHEA, EPA and glutathione are also helpful. Be careful though, excessive intake of some nutrients (like zinc) can actually suppress immunity. Glyconutrients found in shiitake/maitake mushrooms and transfer factors are also valuable.

"I no longer take allergy medication"

"When I began drinking noni juice, the main health problems I dealt with at the time were monthly migraines brought on by my menstrual cycle and hayfever. . . . Since drinking 1–2 ounces of noni juice for approximately twenty months, I only get about three migraines a year now. Their severity and duration is greatly decreased.

This spring is the first spring in about thirty years I can actually be glad the season is here and enjoy its beauty. For the first time, I no longer take allergy medication, and I can enjoy being outside. This is fantastic for me. I used to be absolutely miserable in the spring with a runny nose and itchy eyes. Even my eight-year-old son, who has, like me, suffered with hayfever his entire life, is medicine-free this spring.

I'm so thankful for noni juice and how it has improved my quality of life. Everyone in my family drinks noni juice, including my five-year-old daughter, and my three-month-old puppy. . . .

I never want to suffer with debilitating migraines or hayfever like I did before noni juice entered my life. I will never be without it."

Carrie D., USA

Exercise. Exercise increases blood flow, boosts the body's endorphin and serotonin levels, and enhances growth hormone and T-cell production. Research shows that regular exercisers sleep better and are less depressed. In fact a 2001 study in the *Journal of Occupational and Environmental Medicine* from the American College of Occupational and Environmental Medicine found a link between exercise frequency and illness-related absenteeism. When individuals who did not exercise were compared with individuals who exercised one to seven days a week, nonexercising individuals were found to have higher absences than exercisers, even those exercising just one day a week. Two days of aerobic exercise per week was found to be more favorable than one, but no difference was found between individuals exercising four or more times a week compared with those working out more than one day a week. This study shows that even two days of aerobic exercise per week may enhance the immune system and ward off illness. Another 2001 study found that men who started moderate to regular exercise training later in life may possibly suffer from less age-related decline in immune system function—specifically T-cell function and innate immunity.

Plus, a 2002 AIDS patient care journal for nurses reviewed the use of certain types of exercise to counteract involuntary weight loss associated with the HIV virus. Called AIDS wasting syndrome (AWS), the condition is a serious complication of the virus that can compromise health. However, many studies have found exercise useful for the treatment and prevention of this side effect.

Diet. Not eating a balanced diet can deprive you of nutrients essential for optimal immune function, but equally detrimental are the preservatives, chemicals, sugar, bad fats and empty calories you may be consuming. Artificial elements in your food may be putting stress on your body and your immune system, especially if consumed in excess, and eating too much sugar leaves you more susceptible to infection.

In Dr. Michael B. Schachter's book *Food, Mind and Mood*, he suggests that certain individuals may develop food sensitivities to specific foods. The body responds to these sensitivities by producing antibodies resulting in food allergies. Food allergies can range from mild to severe, but no matter how insignificant they may seem, they still add more to your immune system's workload and may potentially weaken your immunity against disease.

Sleep. Good sleep is essential for a healthy immune system. As mentioned in the last chapter, it is important to establish a regular schedule for retiring in the evening and waking in the morning. A bedtime routine may help you relax after a stressful day. Adequate sleep is essential for the body to recharge and function properly. Chronic sleep deprivation compromises not only the immune system, but possibly many other essential bodily functions.

Relax. If you are overwhelmed with responsibilities, consider doing daily meditation. Meditation can alter brain function, improving endocrine function and enhancing immune function. Dr. Andrew Weil has an excellent meditation compact disc geared especially for using meditation to improve health. If meditation is not your thing, try simple breathing exercises or take a stress management class. The negative effects of chronic stress are severe and should not be ignored.

Complementary herbs: echinacea, goldenseal, olive leaf, grapefruit seed extract (GSE), garlic, ashwagandha, astragalus, aloe vera, elderberry

CHAPTER SIX

The Cancer Connection

• Common medical treatments for cancer	• Noni's anticancer substances
	• Cancer studies using noni
• Noni's potential for cell disease	• Other cancer fighting methods

In the previous chapter, I talked about cancerous tumors as one result of immune dysfunction. Cancer has been around for centuries (despite efforts to attribute it solely to modern industrialized societies). References are made to it in ancient texts, and early human remains confirm its long existence, although it wasn't officially defined until the 1800s. In fact, cancer cells (mutated or malignant cells) are produced by the body every day, but they are usually eliminated by immune cells. A cancer cell loses its "self marker" (which identifies it as the body's own cell), so that it can be destroyed. When the body fails to recognize and get rid of cancer cells they spread and tumors develop.

Cell by mutated cell, cancer conquers one organ and moves to the next, feeding on the organ's energy supplies, until it spreads so much that its victim cannot survive. All it takes is one diseased cell that avoids detection by the immune system and begins to replicate. The reasons behind this immune system breakdown aren't completely understood and some speculate that cancer is more common now than it used to be.

Scientists predict that approximately one in three Americans will have cancer sometime in their lives.

Because of funding and research, your chances of surviving cancer are much greater than they used to be even though the number of cancer cases hasn't declined. Modern medicine has helped a great deal in the fight against cancer by finding methods for early diagnosis, and cancer treatments have also progressed in amazing ways in recent years. Today scientists have a better understanding of how cancer works and how the body defends against it. Excluding lung cancer, overall cancer deaths are currently down by about 15 percent.

Still, considering how far cancer research and treatment has advanced in the last fifty or more years, one would think that cancer would be less of a threat than it is. One explanation for cancer's continued prominence is the fact that in general, people are living longer. Your risk of getting cancer increases as you age because each day you are exposed to thousands of carcinogenic (cancer-causing) substances. Simply stated, the longer you live, the more carcinogens you are exposed to over a lifetime. Only one renegade cancer cell needs to fool your immune system for you to potentially develop cancer. Plus, as mentioned in **Chapter 1**, Americans as a whole are not eating right or exercising enough for optimal health. These and other lifestyle factors may make us more susceptible to illnesses—including cancer.

No one can deny the importance of traditional medicine for those diagnosed with cancer, but many people have decided that alternative medicine offers a great way to reduce their cancer risk or augment traditional cancer treatments. A good diet, regular exercise and nutritional supplements combined with meditation and other mind-body treatments can create an effective anticancer, whole-health plan. The American Cancer Society's *Cancer Prevention and Early Detection Facts and Figures 2002* states, "For the majority of Americans who do not use tobacco products [considered one of the biggest cancer risks], dietary choices and physical activity are the most important modifiable determinants of cancer risk. Nutritional factors account for about one-third of U.S. cancer deaths." Clearly physical activity and proper nutrition are essential to reducing cancer risk and boosting immune power.

The nutritional and immune boosting capabilities of noni may provide a valuable complement to any health plan, including cancer prevention diets. But before we discuss the proven effects of noni on cancer cells, let's take a quick look at traditional cancer treatments.

COMMON MEDICAL TREATMENTS FOR CANCER

Given the scope and limitations of this book, I cannot possibly cover every cancer treatment available. There are numerous types of cancer, and each requires a specific set of therapies. Treatment options are also determined by how early the cancer is detected, where it is located and many other factors. The following is a summary of the most common major cancer treatments.

Surgery

As the oldest cancer treatment, surgery is used at various stages in cancer treatment (and diagnosis), and due to medical advances, it is often successful for many types of cancer. Ideally, surgery is meant to remove cancerous tumors and keep the body functioning as normally as possible. In fact, surgery offers the greatest chance for a cancer cure in many patients. In fact, most individuals diagnosed with cancer will undergo some type of surgical procedure. Surgery is most effective for those in early stages of the disease.

Surgical procedures for cancer usually accomplish one or more specific goals. Some individuals undergo preventive surgery before they get cancer. Precancerous tissues (prone to malignancy) are removed in order to prevent tumors from ever occurring. This procedure is often done in individuals with colon polyps, precancerous skin conditions or those with an inherited risk—like those diagnosed with what is being called the "breast cancer gene" (BRCA1 or BRCA2).

Other surgeries (often called biopsies) are used to diagnose cancer by obtaining a tissue sample. The sample is looked at under a microscope in order to determine if it is cancerous. If a biopsy shows that the cells are cancerous, a "staging surgery" may be done to determine how advanced the cancer is and how much it has spread. One type of staging surgery is called a laparoscopy, where a small camera is attached to a tube and inserted in the abdomen wall. Supportive surgeries are frequently used to help the effectiveness of other treatments. For example, a catheter port could be surgically placed under the skin so that chemotherapy treatments can be administered. Finally, tumor removal, the primary treatment for early stages of cancer, is referred to as "curative surgery." Tumor removal is used when the cancer is confined to one (operable) area, and there is a good chance that doctors can remove all of the cancerous tissue.

A cancer patient may also receive other types of surgery that do not diagnose or remove the cancer, like reconstructive surgery for breast cancer patients, which is meant to help the patient restore their appearance. Other restorative procedures help recover body functions, such as prosthetics used after oral cavity cancer surgeries. Some surgeries are used for advanced cancer patients. They do not cure the cancer patient, but rather help deal with cancer complications that cause pain or disability.

Radiation Therapy

Radiation therapy, also called *radiotherapy* and *irradiation*, is a common cancer treatment used in over half of all cancer cases, including breast, lung, prostate and brain cancers. In fact, some cancer patients only need radiation therapy to beat cancer entirely.

Radiation therapy basically consists of high-energy wave treatments using x-rays, gamma rays, or even electrons or protons to destroy cancerous cells. Many doctors use radiation to help shrink tumors before an operation so that they can be more easily removed. Radiation can also be used after surgery to ensure that all cancer growth is stopped, in case any cells remain after the tumor is removed.

How does it work? Because cancer cells divide more quickly than normal cells, preventing them from multiplying is very important. Radiation therapy delivers high dosage radiation to cancerous tumors. The radiation damages or kills cancer cells so they cannot divide and spread. Normal cells may also be affected by radiation, but these cells recover over time. Radiation therapy can be delivered externally or internally and is aimed only at cancerous tissue; whereas, chemotherapy delivers its treatment to the entire body.

Side effects of radiation therapy vary depending on the kind of cancer and radiation used and include fatigue, dry, itchy or peeling skin, inflammation in the mouth, memory loss, decreased sex drive, intolerance to cold, radiation necrosis, shortness of breath, coughing, nausea, vomiting, diarrhea, infertility, erectile dysfunction, vaginal bleeding and secondary cancers.

Chemotherapy

Chemotherapy, or "chemo" as it is sometimes called, is simply the use of drugs to treat cancer. There are more than one hundred types of chemotherapy drugs, and they are usually used in combination (called *combination chemotherapy*), rather than alone. This is because each drug has a different effect in the body, and so the drugs are combined for all the desired effects necessary to fight a particular form of cancer.

Combining the drugs also reduces the likelihood of building a resistance to them, which would make them less effective.

Chemotherapy works by destroying cancer cells, in the original tumor and in cancer cells that may have spread throughout the body, depending on how advanced the cancer is. Specific drug combinations, dosages, timing, frequency and the duration of treatment will vary from person to person. The goals of chemotherapy, however, are simple: The treatment is meant to slow cancer growth and keep cancer cells from spreading to healthy tissue, as well as relieving the accompanying symptoms. Ultimately, chemotherapy may cure your cancer, depending on what kind of cancer you have and how advanced it is.

Many times chemo is used in combination with surgery and/or radiation therapy. When it is used prior to surgery it's called *neoadjuvant therapy* and post surgery chemo is called *adjuvant therapy*.

Side effects of chemotherapy include nausea, vomiting, hair loss, fatigue, and increased susceptibility to bruising, bleeding and infection. Chemo side effects are notorious for being unpleasant; however, most people experience only one or two side effects, and the severity of these varies from person to person. Some side effects will also ease over time or may be relieved with other medications.

Immunotherapy

A relatively new approach to cancer therapy works with the immune system by using antibodies specially designed to recognize specific cancer cells. Scientists are able to obtain these antibodies by using hybridoma technology. A hybridoma is produced when specific antigens are injected into mice, and then antibodies are collected and fused with cancerous immune cells. Once a hybridoma cell is formed, it can be cloned and tested until an effective antibody is produced. These antibodies work with natural toxins, drugs or radioactive substances to seek their targeted cancer cells and destroy them. Toxins can also be attached to immune cells called lymphokines (disease-fighting white blood cells) and sent to cells with receptors for the improved lymphokine fighters.

Complementary and alternative medicine also believes in treatments that work with the immune system. One treatment that is gaining popularity among cancer patients who use CAM therapies is noni supplementation.

NONI'S POTENTIAL FOR CELL DISEASE

Cancer starts at the cellular level. By now you are probably familiar with xeronine, a compound produced by the body that promotes cell health. It is believed that noni prompts the production of this and other compounds that repair abnormal cells and keep normal cells healthy. In fact, multiple compounds in noni are believed to enhance or strengthen immune function by stimulating anticancer activity in the body's own defense system. For instance, cells called interleukins, messenger cells for the immune system, are stimulated by noni supplementation. Interleukins are necessary to activate immune fighters like natural killer cells, B cells and T lymphocytes. In fact, interleukin-4 cells are believed to interfere with cancer cell growth. One type of interferon, which activates macrophages, is also stimulated by noni compounds. Macrophages are important to cancer research because they secrete a substance called tumor necrosis factor that kills malignant cells. Noni is also believed to enhance the production and activity of natural killer cells, some of the most powerful immune cells.

The best way to discuss noni's potential is to discuss each anticancer substance separately. You will notice that these compounds have been mentioned before, but this section will discuss their impact on cancer.

"I found out I had a tumor in my throat"

"I started taking noni when I became seriously ill. I found out I had a tumor in my throat that was putting pressure on my 4th and 5th vertebrae. I couldn't breath out of my nose at all. . . .I didn't have insurance . . . I took some money I was saving and purchased noni juice. I started drinking it and . . . the tumor drained. My stiff neck went away for good. My headaches that I had experienced for ten years are gone. . . .I have no more back-aches. The pain in my arm and fingers went away after a few weeks. My hands and feet are no longer freezing.

I can breath and I'm pain free. Noni is not a cure at all, but it can help . . . I have energy that I haven't had since I was in my twenties. I sleep better. I have no more acid reflux. I feel 99 percent better. . . .

Just the other day I did a breast exam, and I discovered that the hardness around my breast was gone. . . . For years I just lived with that pain because I knew that it wasn't cancer, until today. I checked my breast and it's all gone. . . . My husband drinks noni now, and it has lowered his blood pressure. We will always drink noni."

Drucilla B., USA

NONI'S ANTICANCER SUBSTANCES

Proxeronine: A chemical in noni called proxeronine is thought to stimulate the production of xeronine in the body. As just mentioned, xeronine positively affects cell function, promoting normal function in healthy cells and restoring it in abnormal cells (such as cancer cells). In the chapter on immune function, xeronine was listed as having positive effects on various immune cells, which research has borne out. These findings may be critical to theories about cancer prevention.

Ursolic Acid: Found in noni leaf, ursolic acid is classified as a chemopreventive agent. Scientific trials have looked into its effects on prostate and breast cancer cells with promising results. Ursolic acid appears to program cancer cells to self-destruct. It also positively affects immune function in general. The next section will discuss ursolic acid in more detail.

Nitric Oxide: Noni is believed to promote the production of nitric oxide in the body. Earlier in this book, I discussed the essential and varied roles of nitric oxide in promoting health. It is known to regulate blood pressure and fight cardiovascular diseases and microbial infection. Another benefit of nitric oxide is seen in the treatment of cancer. Because it enhances immune cell activity (like macrophages) it can fight off not only cold and flu viruses, but tumors as well. How? Noni experts believe that it interferes with the DNA synthesis of dangerous cells, causing them to self-destruct.

Damnacanthal: Damnacanthal is believed to block or inhibit the cellular function of RAS cells, which are considered pre-cancerous cells. Research has shown noni's powerful effects on cancerous malignancies, and many believe that damnacanthal accounts for part of noni's cancer-fighting properties. How does it work? Basically, damnacanthal "convinces" cancer cells that they are healthy, which halts or slows down cell multiplication and cancer growth. This compound has proven useful on lung, colon and pancreatic cancer, as well as leukemia, and future testing may prove its usefulness against other cancers. The next section has more information on damnacanthal.

CANCER STUDIES USING NONI

• *Preventing Cancer with Noni.* In 1999, researchers at the Department of Biochemistry at Chiba University, Japan, found that damnacanthal, a compound in noni root, inhibited an enzyme called tyrosine kinase when isolated. Tyrosine kinase helps to promote the growth of malignant cells. Abnormal cells that were treated with damnacanthal prior to ultraviolet light exposure were more rapidly destroyed, illustrating that noni root constituents can stop the activity of tyrosine kinase. Some of the most powerful chemotherapy drugs used today to treat cancer are designed to do the same thing. Noni's damnacanthal content also contributes to programmed malignant cell death, which works to regulate tumor cell growth. In light of this data, damnacanthal from noni may not only prevent cancer, but also be of benefit if you already have cancer.

Moreover, a 2001 issue of *Cancer Research* also reported that two glycosides found in noni juice are cancer protective. The study looked at the juice's effects on cell transformation in mice, and its findings look promising. In fact, the National Institutes of Health (NIH) gave a $300,000 grant to Cancer Research Center of Hawaii in 2001 to test noni in humans.

• *Ursolic Acid and Cancer.* Ursolic acid (found in noni leaf) has been classified as a natural chemopreventive agent. Recent scientific trials testing this powerful acid have confirmed its ability to inhibit a number of cellular changes in (human) breast cells that can cause the growth of cancerous tumors. Ursolic acid suppressed the negative effect of a carcinogenic agent on breast cells in these tests. Another study found that ursolic acid inhibited the growth of a dangerous form of cancer made up of fibrosarcoma cells. And a 2000 issue of the *International Journal of Oncology* investigated the effect of ursolic acid on the growth of (human) prostate cells and found it promoted the elimination of potentially malignant cells. In other words, ursolic acid helped program cancer cells to self-destruct.

• *Cancer and Noni Fruit.* A 1994 study involving top scientist Anne Hirazumi, Ph.D., cited the anticancer activity of noni compounds against lung cancer. A team of scientists from the University of Hawaii tested the medicinal properties of noni against Lewis lung carcinomas that were artificially transferred to lung tissue in mice. Untreated mice died within twelve days, but mice give noni juice daily lived significantly longer—half lived more than fifty days. Researchers concluded that the chemical constituents of noni juice indirectly enhanced the ability of the immune system to deal with the invading malignancy by boosting macrophage or lymphocyte activity, and even activating certain macrophages to attack. Further evaluation theorized that noni fruit also enhanced T-cell activity, a reaction that may explain the multi-faceted use of noni to treat a variety of infectious diseases.

Further tests using various noni preparations found that mice with lung carcinomas that were treated with concentrated noni lived much longer than mice in the control group, some over 100 percent longer, and 32 percent of mice fed concentrated noni were completely cured. Researchers believe that noni's success was due in part to its stimulation of nitric oxide and interleukins. They also believe that noni could enhance the effectiveness of some anti-cancer drugs while reducing their side effects.

• *Noni May Prevent Malignancies.* In Japan, studies on damnacanthal, a compound in noni fruit, found that it was able to inhibit the function of K-RAS-NRK cells, which are considered precursors to certain cancerous malignancies. Noni plant extract was added to RAS cells , which were then incubated. Observations of noni supported the belief that noni was able to significantly inhibit RAS cellular function. Among 500 plant extracts tested, noni was determined to be most effective against RAS cells. Its damnacanthal content was clinically described in 1993 as "a new inhibitor of RAS function." Scientists at the Department of Pharmacology at the John A. Burns School of Medicine in Honolulu also reported in 1996 that noni's ability to modulate or boost the immune system also contributes to its anticancer activity. A study from the University of Illinois College of Medicine also found that noni could reduce incidences of cancer in mice exposed to carcinogenic agents. Specifically, researchers noted protective effects on the liver, kidneys, heart and lungs.

OTHER CANCER FIGHTING METHODS

Nutritional Supplements. Earlier I mentioned that your body is exposed to thousands of carcinogens each day. Antioxidants found in lycopene, grape seed extract, green tea, soy, vitamins C and E and beta carotene rid the body of free radicals, which are dangerous cellular by-products of our environment. Antioxidants can also lower cancer risk. Cancer patients may have difficulty consuming or absorbing the necessary amounts of nutrients they need. A daily multivitamin and mineral is imperative to counteract cancer, especially during its treatment phase.

Exercise. To prevent cancer it is imperative that you stay physically active (or start now) and strive to maintain a healthy weight—being over- or underweight is a health risk. Strive to exercise at least thirty minutes (or more) every day. Staying moderately active not only gives you energy and helps you deal with stress, it also can protect you from disease. You don't even have to do thirty minutes of exercise all at one time, according to some experts. You can break it up into ten or fifteen minute increments—or whatever works for you.

Anything that makes you breathe hard is considered moderate activity: a brisk walk, gardening, riding a bike, washing a car, rigorous housecleaning, dancing and sex. While you're watching television, you can spend some time lifting small weights and doing stretches. What's important is that you work daily exercise into your regular routine so it becomes a lifetime habit.

If you have been diagnosed with cancer and are undergoing treatment, starting and maintaining an exercise program can be difficult. Fatigue, pain and nausea can be discouraging and troublesome. Not everyone should exercise, depending on how advanced their condition is. You should consult with a doctor before beginning any program. How rigorous your routine is will depend on both your current condition and how active and healthy you were before you got sick. If you are able to exercise, make sure that you schedule in times for rest and relaxation so that you may adequately recuperate. If your energy levels fall too low, you may have to skip your next scheduled routine or you may lose your motivation, so take it easy!

Your doctor will be able to tell you if some types of exercise should be added or deleted from your routine, depending on your health and potential risks. If you were a regular exerciser before getting cancer, maintaining that routine may be therapeutic because it proves that some areas of your life remain unchanged despite your illness. Still, check with a doctor about the safety of continuing your current program.

Diet. Eating a balanced diet is particularly important for individuals undergoing treatment for cancer and those at risk for or recovering from cancer. Individuals with cancer may find their appetite has been affected by the illness and accompanying treatments. Moreover, their condition may also alter the way nutrients are absorbed and used by the body. Some food intolerances may surface as well. Specific nutrient needs will vary from person to person, but eating a variety of foods is essential to boost your strength and energy levels. In addition, a well-balanced diet reduces your risk of secondary infections, enhances your healing ability and helps you better tolerate side effects. The following are imperative to any cancer diet:

- **Water.** Water is essential to good health. Consuming too little could leave you more prone to diarrhea and vomiting if you have cancer and are undergoing treatment.
- **Protein.** Protein is necessary for tissue repair and for normal immune function. It helps you fight infections and recover faster from illness and surgery. Cancer patients need more protein that usual. Good sources include lean meats, poultry, fish, dairy, legumes and nuts and seeds. Soy is a great source of vegetable protein.
- **Carbohydrates.** Carbs should be the source of most of your calories. The amount a person needs depends on their age, weight and how physically active they are. The key to choosing carbohydrates is picking natural over processed, i.e. whole-wheat bread over white, fruits and veggies over sugar products, etc. Fruits, vegetables, grains, beans, pastas, breads and cereals are all good sources of carbohydrates. Broccoli, carrots, asparagus, onion and tomatoes are great choices for the cancer conscious individual. Eating a variety of fruits and vegetables will provide you will the full spectrum of phytonutrients necessary to prevent cancer.
- **Fats.** Not all fat is bad for you. In fact, good fats like those found in nuts, fish and oils like olive oil are crucial to good health—in small amounts. Limit your fat intake and choose good fats over saturated and animal-based fats like butter.

The American Institute for Cancer Research (AICR) has guidelines on nutritious eating to prevent cancer, as well as research updates, recipes and free publications for good health to help you reduce your cancer risk, deal with diagnosed cancer and live a healthier life. Visit **www. aicr.org** or call (800) 843-8114 for more information. The American Cancer Society also has valuable nutrition information (**www.cancer.org** or 1-800-ACS-2345).

Combating Stress. Needless to say, being diagnosed with cancer is a source of enormous stress. Besides worrying about your own mortality and the effects of cancer on your mind and body, you also have to worry about fitting in medical treatments, dealing with side effects, and finding the money to pay for your treatment. You must also handle the extra strain it puts on many of your relationships, as well as maintaining your normal responsibilities. Fighting off the damaging effects of stress is very important, because stress leaves you more vulnerable to depression and can interfere with immune function and your ability to recover.

One way to combat the negative effects of stress is to join or form a support community where you can discuss the effects of your illness and ways to deal with it. Your community may consist of friends and family, or you may want to consider joining a support community for individuals with cancer. Meditation and yoga may also help you deal with your new stresses. Both positively affect brain function and boost immunity.

Complementary herbs: astragalus, chlorella, cordyceps sinesis, garlic, green tea, pau d'arco, transfer factor, red clover, maitake, shiitake and reishi mushrooms

CHAPTER SEVEN

Noni: The Answer to Cardiovascular Disease

- High blood pressure: what is it and how does it happen?
- Health problems caused by high blood pressure
- What can be done about hypertension?
- Using noni for high blood pressure
- Preventing hypertension
- Preventing a stroke
- Heart disease: how you can fight the number one killer
- What causes coronary artery disease?
- Heart protective habits

Almost sixty-two million Americans currently suffer from at least one type of cardiovascular disease (CVD)—about one in five adults. Fifty million of these sufferers are diagnosed with high blood pressure, another 12.6 million with heart disease, and over 4.5 million have suffered a stroke. In addition, nearly five million have some degree of congestive heart failure.

Approximately one in every 2.5 deaths is caused by cardiovascular disease, and that number is even greater (nearly 60 percent) when figures include cardiovascular disease as a contributing factor in addition to the primary cause of death. In fact, since 1900, cardiovascular disease has been the number one killer in the United States every year except 1918. And in recent years, it has taken more lives than the next seven leading causes of death combined. Experts estimate that about two people die every minute from some form of CVD, and they calculate that life expectancy would increase by about seven years if all forms of CVD were eliminated.

In response to these startling facts, organizations like the American Heart Association have endeavored to increase public awareness about cardiovascular diseases, their risk factors and what can be done to prevent them. Still, cardio-vascular-related deaths have actually increased in recent years. A discouraging fact when you realize that many forms of cardiovascular disease are largely preventable with regular exercise, a heart-healthy diet and other healthy habits (like not smoking).

Even by incorporating healthy lifestyles, you still may be at risk for cardiovascular disease. For this reason, taking dietary supplements like noni can enhance your heart-health strategy, and may further reduce your risk of developing high blood pressure, heart disease and stroke. Noni's heart benefits, especially for hypertension, will be the subject of this chapter, but first, here's a refresher course on what hypertension is.

HIGH BLOOD PRESSURE: WHAT IS IT AND HOW DOES IT HAPPEN?

High blood pressure, or hypertension, is a preventable condition that affects about one in four Americans and can lead to more serious illnesses (i.e. stroke, heart or kidney disease) and even death. In fact, more people across the globe take medication for high blood pressure than for any other health condition. Actually, high blood pressure is a risk factor more than a disease. It is a sign that you are having circulatory system problems—much like sneezing may be a sign of a cold or allergies. Rising blood pressure levels are a sign that the heart is having to pump harder to move blood through the circulatory system.

Many experts believe that high blood pressure is largely the result of lifestyle and diet since most cases of hypertension occur in industrialized nations like the United States. Incidences of high blood pressure in Third World countries are far lower. Most people have primary or essential hypertension, and its exact cause often remains a mystery. For a few individuals, however, the cause can be attributed pregnancy, birth control pills, hormones, tumors, or kidney disease. This type of high blood pressure is called secondary hypertension. Primary hypertension is incurable, but secondary hypertension can be treated (or reversed) if its cause is identified.

Hypertension risk also increases with age; about half of Americans over the age of sixty-five are diagnosed with it. Certain minority groups like African Americans are more likely to develop hypertension, and individuals with diabetes and other health problems may also have a higher risk for the disease. Postmenopausal women, smokers and individuals living in southern states like Mississippi, Louisiana and Alabama (also called the "Stroke Belt States") are more likely candidates for high blood pressure as well. Heredity may also play a role, but regardless of your risk factors (or lack thereof), no one should assume they are either immune or doomed to hypertension. It is also important to remember that there are no warning signs or symptoms for hypertension, so it is imperative to have your blood pressure checked regularly and to take preventive measures.

A Closer Look at the Circulatory System

Problems with the circulatory system are no small matter. Through a network of veins, arteries and capillaries, this system delivers not only oxygen and nutrients, but also hormones, immune substances and other vital chemicals to virtually every cell in the body. It also aids in waste product removal, maintains body temperature, and balances water and electrolyte levels. Knowing all of this, it is easy to see why problems with the circulatory system are associated with some of the top causes of death in the United States and abroad.

The circulatory system is made up of the heart and blood and lymph vessels, responsible for moving blood and lymph through the body. (The lymphatic system is discussed in more detail in **Chapter 5**.) Consider for a moment that the average adult has approximately five quarts of blood in his body, and that this blood makes its way through the entire body about once every minute, meaning that each day, a healthy heart deals with *over 7,000 quarts of blood.*

Various factors mediate the speed of blood flow, including heart rate and force, as well as the health of the veins. Blood vessels called arteries carry the blood from the heart to body tissues. Blood pressure actually refers to the force (or pressure) of that blood as it pushes against artery walls. With every heartbeat, blood leaves the heart and is pumped into those vessels by the contraction of the heart muscles. Your blood pressure is highest at this moment (systolic pressure). In between contractions, when your heart rests, your blood pressure falls (diastolic pressure). Both of these numbers make up your total blood pressure reading and are usually written as a fraction (i.e. 120/80 mm Hg), where the top number is your systolic pressure and the bottom is diastolic pressure. The letters "mm Hg" refers to millimeters of mercury, because the original blood pressure gauges used mercury. We use the same measure today but use air instead of mercury to measure blood pressure now.

Blood Pressure: What Is Healthy and What Isn't?

Of course, not all changes in blood pressure are bad. In a healthy individual, variations are normal. Your blood pressure will rise when you go jogging and fall when you are at rest. In fact, your blood pressure reading is often slightly higher than usual when taken at a doctor's office because your body is responding to the stress of the situation. Most experts agree that optimal blood pressure for a healthy heart (eighteen years and older) should be below 120/80 mm Hg, but under 140/90 mm Hg is considered normal but borderline. Individuals with blood pressure over 160/100 mm Hg are in the danger zone, and those with a reading over 180/110 mm Hg are in the highest risk group. Although considered dangerous in the past, below-average blood pressure is no longer considered a health risk by medical practitioners.

Blood pressure only becomes unhealthy when it stays high the majority of the time. As a result, artery walls are constantly under above-average pressure, and if not corrected, this condition eventually leads to other problems, like arteriosclerosis or hardened arteries. The damaged vessels then collect fats and cholesterol, which restrict blood flow eventually causing a stroke or heart attack if left untreated. Ultimately, if left untreated, chronically high blood pressure will weaken arteries, making them more vulnerable to ruptures and cholesterol plaque build up. When this happens, inordinate amounts of strain are placed on the heart.

HEALTH PROBLEMS CAUSED BY HIGH BLOOD PRESSURE

Enlarged Heart. Because hypertension causes your heart to work overtime, it can sustain damage. If left untreated, heart muscle becomes thicker and stretches, resulting in abnormal functioning and eventually, in fluid accumulation in the lungs.

Heart Attack. High blood pressure can lead to vessel blockages and subsequent narrowing. When arteries are blocked, blood flow is reduced and the heart becomes oxygen deprived, resulting in angina or chest pain. A heart attack occurs when blood flow to the heart is completely cut off.

Stroke. Build up in the arteries caused by hypertension can also restrict blood flow to the brain. If one of these blood vessels breaks or if a blood clot forms that blocks one of these narrowed arteries, a stroke occurs. Strokes caused by broken vessels are *hemorrhagic strokes*, and those caused by a clot are called *thrombotic strokes*.

Kidney Disease. Arteriosclerosis can also affect vessels in the kidneys. The kidneys filter waste products from the blood. When kidney blood vessels are restricted, the organ becomes less effective in ridding the body of waste. This allows toxins to stay in the blood, which can result in kidney damage and subsquent kidney failure. The only solutions once this happens are a kidney transplant or dialysis.

WHAT CAN BE DONE ABOUT HYPERTENSION?

Research on risk groups has yielded many answers on how to prevent and treat high blood pressure. High fat, high cholesterol diets may increase your risk of developing hypertension, as can diets high in salt and refined foods. Regular exercise reduces your risk, as does maintaining a healthy weight. Health experts have developed guidelines to lower your risk of developing high blood pressure (which are also good for those already diagnosed):

- Limit your intake of alcoholic beverages and don't smoke.
- Choose heart-healthy foods and limit your fat and salt intake.
- Engage in aerobic exercise on a regular basis, preferable thirty minutes a day.
- Maintain a healthy weight for your height and frame. If you are overweight, make losing weight a top priority.

Doctors will typically prescribe medication for anyone with chronic hypertension. For those interested in complementary therapies, there are a number of herbs and supplements that can also help you win the battle against hypertension. Potentially beneficial herbs include ginseng and garlic along with coenzyme Q10. Noni also offers a number of potential benefits for anyone suffering from high blood pressure.

USING NONI FOR HIGH BLOOD PRESSURE

As previously mentioned, one of noni's traditional applications is treating high blood pressure. In fact, recent research on noni's chemical compounds and their effects supports this use. Furthermore, because noni is an adaptogenic plant and regulates both high and low blood pressure with little or no side effects, it is much safer than many prescriptions. Moreover, if you take noni for hypertension, you are likely to experience many other health benefits. How many prescription drugs can do that? Keep in mind that the whole noni plant including its roots, bark, leaves, and fruit can be used together for maximum synergistic effect. Let's take a closer look at three compounds that give noni its ability to regulate blood pressure.

Nitric Oxide. Although noni does not contain nitric oxide, it promotes its production in the body. The many health applications of nitric oxide have already been discussed in earlier chapters, but let me quickly review it benefits for those with hypertension. Studies on nitric oxide have found that it may lower blood pressure by encouraging blood vessel elasticity, which ultimately alleviates undue stress on arteries and the heart. Experts believe that nitric oxide may be released by the body into the bloodstream to regulate blood pressure by relaxing artery walls. In fact, many studies have used nitric oxide therapy to treat hypertension because it not only dilates vessels, but

"I was listed in critical condition"

"My name is Glenn, and on July 15, 1995, I experienced a heart attack. On July 20, 1995, I underwent open-heart surgery for a double bypass. Complications forced me to undergo a second surgery. I remained on a life support system for the next five days on a touch and go basis. Finally, after one month I was released from the hospital. On three different occasions I was rushed to the emergency room due to more complications, each time I was listed in critical condition.

After heart surgery, doctors prescribed seven different medications for me. Today I no longer need any! Not only did noni juice allow me to be free of prescription drugs, it has lowered my blood pressure, relieved my carpel tunnel, improved my eyesight . . . helped me beat skin cancer . . . and relieved prostrate problems.

The doctors said I would never be able to go back to work again and would be on disability for the rest of my life because of my heart. I will be seventy years young this year, and I am back to work as a stonemason. I am so thankful for what noni juice has done for me."

Glenn L., USA

also discourages blood clotting. University of Hawaii studies have noted that noni appears to enhance nitric oxide production and encourage the opening of constricted blood vessels.

Scopoletin. Experts in noni research agree that one compound in noni, scopoletin, is at the heart of its blood pressure regulating power. Studies on the isolated compound show an abundance of evidence supporting its antihypertensive effects. Some critics believe that scopoletin is so powerful that it may even take blood pressure to dangerous lows. Keep in mind that the only documented cases of this effect only occurred when using the isolated compound. When scopoletin is taken as a part of the noni plant and not as an isolated supplement, it does not render this effect. In fact, it appears to normalize low blood pressure as well. The mechanism behind this remarkable action is due to the extraordinary array of medicinal compounds found in noni that work together in ways that would not be possible if isolated.

Xeronine. A discussion of blood pressure would not be complete without mentioning the benefits of xeronine on hypertension. Although noni contains no xeronine, it does contain proxeronine, a chemical that is believed to enhance xeronine production in the body. As mentioned in previous chapters, xeronine normalizes cellular reactions and encourages proper cell function. Because hardened artery walls are comprised of damaged cells, the cell-repairing properties of xeronine may help to reverse the disease. Furthermore, if noni is taken as a preventive measure against high blood pressure, xeronine enhancement may help to keep the circulatory system healthy by preventing cholesterol build-up in the first place. Certainly enhanced levels of xeronine would also benefit those with heart disease, stroke, kidney disease or an enlarged heart. I will discuss heart disease and stroke in more detail later in this chapter.

PREVENTING HYPERTENSION

Because most cases of hypertension are considered incurable by the medical community, preventing it is the best course of action for healthy individuals. Noni is an excellent supplement to include in your disease prevention strategy and works best when combined with these recommendations:

Stop smoking. (As if there aren't enough reasons to quit already.) For those of you who haven't been able to kick the

habit, perhaps the heart-stopping effects of tobacco will provide the motivation to give it another try.

Eat heart healthy. The phrase "heart healthy" is becoming
commonplace, as are the American Heart Association
endorsements appearing on many grocery items (i.e. oat-
meal). Heart-conscious eating is more than food labels
though. A diet that emphasizes plenty of fruits and vegetables, whole grains and legumes provides the foundation for
heart health.

Limit your meat consumption, and choose lean meats and
fish over beef. It is a proven fact that vegetarians have lower
risks for heart-related diseases like high blood pressure.
Hypertension prevention also means reducing sugar, salt, saturated fat, caffeine and alcohol intake, while including more
fatty fish (like salmon) and beneficial oils (like olive and
flaxseed) in your diet.

Foods that increase your hypertension risk include smoked
meats, some preservatives and animal products like cheese and
cream. Garlic, onions, celery and pectin-containing fruits may
lower your risk. The American Heart Association has a number
of publications and cookbooks available to help Americans eat
healthier. You can also download *An Eating Plan for Healthy
Americans* without cost from their site. Visit **americanheart.org**
for more information or call 1-800-AHA-USA-1.

Exercise. If you are overweight, start (or restart) an exercise
(and diet) program to take the extra pounds off. There is a
direct relationship between excess body weight and high blood
pressure. That extra weight can make you as much as six times
more likely to develop high blood pressure. It is especially
important to keep a desirable weight if you collect fat in your
midsection (apple shape) instead of your hips (pear shape).
Apple-shaped people are also more likely to develop type-2 diabetes. Even losing a little weight can make a big difference.

It is important to develop a program that you can stick with for life. According to statistics, most individuals stop their exercise program after two months, and those that go longer often drop the program after a year. So make sure to start slow and vary your routine so you don't get bored. Also, some experts recommend starting an exercise program before beginning a diet. Beginning a diet without exercise may leave you sapped of energy and more hungry. You are more likely to see quicker weight-loss results if you begin exercising first, then cut calories.

While running and skiing are incredible calorie burners, swimming, walking, cycling and jogging are great examples of cardiovascular activity. You don't need a gym membership to be healthy—even golfing, gardening and housecleaning burn calories. The important thing is to stay active every day. For those who are especially busy, sneak in aerobic exercise by parking farther away from the store and using stairs instead of elevators whenever possible. Aim for at least thirty minutes of activity each day. If you suffer from health problems, be sure to check with a doctor before starting a rigorous program. Combining an exercise program with stress management may compound and accelerate its health benefits.

Supplements. Antioxidant vitamins C and E are both essential for circulatory system health, as are calcium, magnesium, potassium and selenium. A fiber and a fish oil supplement may also be helpful. Herbs like astragalus, cayenne, chamomile, fennel, ginseng, glucomannan and rosemary may also be beneficial. Before taking any supplement, check for any contraindications. Be aware that some herbs may aggravate hypertension or interfere with hypertensive medications.

The National Heart, Lung and Blood Institute has an education program for preventing hypertension and are an excellent source for further information on avoiding this risky condition. They can be contacted at their website **www.nhlbi.nih.gov** or by calling (301) 496-4236.

PREVENTING A STROKE

One possible side effect of untreated high blood pressure is stroke, currently the third most common cause of death in the United States. Hypertension accounts for at least 70 percent of all strokes. Other risk factors include smoking, diabetes and obesity or inactivity. In addition, individuals over the age of sixty-five, particularly women, are at increased risk for stroke. Even estrogen fluctuations in postmenopausal women appear to be linked to stroke risk. Keep in mind, however, that nearly thirty percent of people under sixty-five will also have a stroke. Some minority groups also have increased risk, as do those who live in southeastern states like Georgia (the "Stroke Belt States").

As mentioned, strokes are caused when a blood vessel bursts (hemorrhagic strokes) or when a blood clot dislodges (thrombotic strokes). Noni's clot-reducing properties make it an excellent supplement for stroke prevention, and anecdotal evidence supports this use. Its effectiveness against strokes is not surprising considering that noni also is used to treat contributing factors to a stroke such as diabetes and hypertension. Interestingly, some individuals have used noni to help them kick addictive habits like smoking and alcoholism, which help reduce the risk of stroke. Aside from preventing high blood pressure, there are other things you can do to reduce your stroke risk:

Stop smoking. Smokers are two to three times more likely to suffer a stroke. The sooner you quit the better, since your stroke risk is elevated for as long as twenty years after quitting.

Limit alcohol and caffeine intake. Moderate intake of alcohol has been linked to decreased stroke risk, but heavy alcohol use has the opposite effect. Caffeine has also been shown to increase the risk of stroke in individuals with high blood pressure. Illegal drugs and steroids have also been linked to an increased stroke risk.

Avoid B vitamin deficiencies. Deficiencies of vitamins B6, B12 and folic acid can lead to dangerously high levels of homocysteine, an amino acid. This condition can lead to heart disease and increased stroke risk. In fact, it is the second leading cause of strokes. Homocysteine appears to have negative effects on artery walls and may make the blood more prone to clotting. B vitamin deficiencies have also been linked to depression and hormone imbalances. It's well known that low folic acid levels can also cause birth defects. Vegetarians should take consider taking a B12 supplement since most sources of the vitamin are in meat products.

Stay fit. Obesity not only raises your blood pressure, but also makes you more vulnerable to type-2 diabetes and high cholesterol. Abdominal fat is especially dangerous. Staying active and maintaining a healthy weight for your frame will reduce your stroke risk.

Keep healthy blood sugar levels. Diabetics are particularly vulnerable to stroke, especially type-2, noninsulin-dependent diabetics. These individuals still produce insulin, but their cells have developed a resistance to it, a condition called hyperinsulinemia. These high insulin levels reduce beneficial cholesterol (HDL) and make the body more vulnerable to blood clots.

Prevent heart disease. Surgical treatments like coronary bypass may increase stroke risk, as do heart attacks and some anti-clotting drugs used in the treatment of heart disease.

Manage stress. Learning to relax is not optional when it comes to a healthy heart. Prolonged periods of stress not only increase your risk of developing hypertension, they also increase your stroke risk (and your chances of dying if you have a second stroke).

Weigh the risks before taking birth control pills. Although low-dose estrogen contraceptives do not seem to increase stroke risk, pills with high levels of estrogen may increase your risk of having a stroke. African American women, smokers, women with hypertension and those who suffer from migraines or clotting disorders should avoid the pill if possible, since their risks are much higher. Women with high blood pressure should avoid contraceptives with progestins as well. Overall, however, the risks are considered small (as little as eight in every 100,000 users).

Treat chronic infections quickly. Some studies have found a link between bacterial and viral infections and some circulatory problems, including stroke. Gum disease and respiratory infections seem to have a significant correlation especially in younger individuals. Noni supplementation may also be helpful in treating infection.

Other risk factors include chronic headaches and migraines, sleep apnea, pregnancy, low testosterone in men, sickle-cell anemia, the presence of (aPL) antibodies in the blood, and the use of some drugs, such as aspirin and some over-the-counter decongestants. If any of these risks apply to you, do what it takes to reduce their effects. Take the necessary precautions to reduce your risk, especially if you have a family history of heart disease, high blood pressure, diabetes or stroke.

Strokes should always be taken seriously. Unlike other cells, brain cells do not be regenerate. Over 150,000 Americans die each year as a result of a stroke (and this number is rising). Although more than half of all victims will live at least five years after their stroke, many suffer from severe complications. It is better to avoid this serious health problem if possible. If you have already suffered from a stroke, don't get discouraged. With the proper lifestyle changes, you can lead a productive life. For more information, contact the American Stroke Association at **www.strokeassociation.org** or call 1-888-4-STROKE.

HEART DISEASE: HOW YOU CAN FIGHT THE NUMBER ONE KILLER

One of the most pervasive and destructive effects of high blood pressure is heart disease, considered a true epidemic in the United States and other developed nations. More than five million Americans are affected by coronary artery disease (CAD) each year, and despite efforts to educate the public and improve treatment, it remains the number one killer by far in many industrialized countries. Moreover, some risk factors for heart disease are inalterable: if you have family history of the disease, you're a postmenopausal woman or a male over the age of forty-five. Despite the grim statistics, there are things that you can do to reduce your risk of developing heart disease, regardless of your risk factors.

WHAT CAUSES CORONARY ARTERY DISEASE?

Heart disease is caused by the narrowing of arteries by plaque (atherosclerosis). Although the chambers of the heart are filled with blood, heart tissue relies on blood vessels on its surface, called coronary arteries, to run properly. There are two coronary arteries on the left side of the heart and one on the right. All three branch out from the aorta. Plaque is made up of fatty substances, proteins, calcium and inflammatory cells that build up over time in the arteries. Fatty deposits can actually begin sticking to vessel walls during preadolescence, and over time in risk-prone individuals, these deposits will interfere with blood flow and eventually cause coronary artery disease. Fatty deposit buildup irritates vessel walls, and in response the body sends a sticky substance to heal itself. This makes vessel walls act like a magnet for other substances like calcium and protein that combine to form plaque. Plaque is characteristically hard on the outside and soft in the middle. If the hard surface cracks or ruptures at all, platelets are send to encourage blood clotting, which further narrows the arteries and restricts blood flow.

In response to a blockage, the body will often develop an alternate form of circulation called collateral circulation where the artery functions by using tiny branches resembling capillaries to bypass the narrowed artery and allow for continued blood flow. Unfortunately, collateral circulation rarely supplies enough blood to tissue especially during times of exertion. As a result, the person may experience heart muscle cramping, referred to as ischemia. Ischemia commonly occurs after eating, with excitement or when exposed to cold temperatures. If ischemia attacks last less than ten minutes, the condition is referred to as stable coronary artery disease.

In other cases, the artery may become totally blocked by plaque, cutting off blood to the heart (called acute coronary syndrome). Three types of CAD fall under this category: unstable angina, myocardial infarction and a heart attack. The type of acute coronary syndrome a person is diagnosed with depends on the amount of time blood flow was stopped and the resulting amount of damage the block created. Acute coronary syndrome can be caused by even a tiny amount of plaque, which is not detectable in a stress test or cardiac catheterization. In some cases, there are no symptoms.

What Are the Symptoms of CAD?

Angina. Commonly referred to as chest pain, this is one of the best indicators of heart disease. The discomfort, heaviness or burning sensation it causes, however, is often mistaken for a less severe complaint—indigestion. Although the pain is usually centered in the chest, the left shoulder and arm may be affected. The pain may also be felt in the jaw and the back.

Palpitations. Also called irregular heartbeats, palpitations may be a sign that something is wrong, especially when your heart beats faster. A panic attack may resemble this heart disease symptom as well, as can certain drug and herb reactions.

Nausea and dizziness. Once again, these symptoms are also common with panic attacks. Check with a doctor either way.

Shortness of breath and abnormal perspiration. These symptoms do not necessarily mean that you have heart disease, but if you are experiencing these things in combination with any of the above, see a doctor immediately. Your doctor will probably ask you about your family history, determine what risk factors you have, and do tests such as an electrocardiogram and an exercise stress test if warranted.

HEART PROTECTIVE HABITS

We have already discussed a number of good habits, including noni supplementation, that can reduce your risk of high blood pressure, a contributing factor for CAD, and stroke. Let's quickly review the best ways to protect your cardiovascular system and your heart. Some of them may sound familiar:

Stop smoking. I've said more than enough on this subject. If you smoke, please find a way to quit for good.

Fight high cholesterol. Beginning a low-fat, low cholesterol diet may not sound appealing, but it can be quite satisfying. You do not have to cut all fat out of your diet, just reduce your fat intake and consume the right kinds of fat. Choose vegetable oils like olive oil over animal fats, and replace some beef and chicken servings with a serving of a fatty fish like salmon. In fact, cutting too much fat (good fat) out of your diet will also have negative effects on your cholesterol (especially good HDL cholesterol).

Exercise! Regular exercise will not only lower your heart disease risk, it can also reduce your risk of diabetes, obesity, high blood pressure, high cholesterol, and chronic stress—all contributing factors for heart disease. Extra pounds mean extra work for your heart.

Control your stress. Failing to regulate stress levels and anger have been found to increase your risk of heart disease. Stress management classes, relaxation exercises and meditation or yoga may be useful.

Begin a heart healthy diet. What does eating heart healthy entail? It means eating plenty of fruits and vegetables, whole grains, and legumes. Limit your meat consumption, and choose lean meats whenever possible. Still confused or don't know where to start? The American Heart Association has a number of cookbooks available to help Americans eat for a healthy heart. You can also download *An Eating Plan for Healthy Americans* for free from their site at **american heart.org** (or call 1-800-AHA-USA-1).

Avoid insulin resistance. Insulin resistance is a common cause of type-2 diabetes, where the body is not able to utilize insulin normally, resulting in abnormal blood sugar levels. Diabetics have an increased risk for heart disease. If you are diabetic, make sure you follow the diet and exercise plan prescribed by your doctor, and take any medications necessary to keep your blood sugar normal. Brittle diabetics (diabetics who suffer from regular blood sugar fluctuations) are particularly susceptible.

Use heart healthy supplements. Noni is a wonderful preventative because of its beneficial effects on the circulatory system. Other beneficial supplements include vitamin E, vitamin C, potassium, calcium and magnesium, garlic, ginger, hawthorne, coenzyme Q10 and essential fatty acids.

CHAPTER EIGHT

Other Uses for Noni

• Asthma	• Digestive problems
• Diabetes	• Pain

So far I have discussed significant ways in which noni supplementation can improve your health, but there are many other illnesses that may be treated with noni. The same properties in noni that affect blood vessels, boost immunity, ease pain and increase energy levels may also combat infections, fight depression and treat digestive, skin and urinary conditions. Although the health problems discussed in this chapter are not the only ones that may benefit from noni supplementation (a more complete list can be found in **Chapter 2**), they are some of the most common. **Chapter 9** also outlines additional uses for noni (such as topical applications of the supplement for burns, cuts and acne, as well as information on using noni to treat a family pet).

ASTHMA

Asthma is a chronic condition experienced by over twelve million people in the United States. It is an incurable, life-threatening upper respiratory problem caused by tightened bronchioles in the lungs. Air flow in these tubes becomes restricted when the tube lining swells or when tightening in surrounding muscle narrows the airways and causes abnormal amounts of mucus to form. The causes for asthma are complex and vary from person to person. We do know it can be triggered by allergens like dust, mold, tobacco smoke or even some food; infections like the common cold; cold air; exercise; medications; stress; air pollution; or chemicals and pesticides.

Asthma cases are actually on the rise in industrialized nations like the United States, and scientists aren't completely sure why. Experts do believe that some individuals may be more vulnerable to developing asthma, especially those with a family history of the illness. Children also have a higher risk of developing asthma, but 30 percent of kids with the disease outgrow it as adults. Allergens are associated more with childhood asthma than attacks experienced by adults.

Mild asthma symptoms include chest tightness, wheezing, coughing and shortness of breath. Severe symptoms, or an asthma attack, consist of breathlessness, inability to talk, blue or gray tinted fingernails, and tight chest muscles and tight neck muscles. For some individuals, even after symptoms end, swelling in the bronchioles can continue for days or weeks, making an individual particularly susceptible to subsequent attacks.

Asthma: Contributing Factors

Scientists believe that individuals with a family history of asthma may be more vulnerable to known triggers of the disease. Genes, however, can't explain all asthma cases or why the number of sufferers continues to increase. Some blame pollution and environmental toxins for the rise, and new links to asthma—like roaches—are being discovered as well. Scientists may not completely understand what sparks an asthma attack, but they do know that repeated inflammatory

asthmatic responses can permanently alter airways both func-
tionally and structurally (called remodeling). Some remodeling offenders include interleukin 13 (mucus producer), neutrophils (white blood cells) and scarring that results from
repeated attacks. Below is a short list of the most common
contributing factors for asthma:

• **Diet.** Food allergies have been linked to asthma. A food
  allergy is an intolerance to a certain food or foods. Other
  symptoms (besides asthma) include hives, mouth irritation,
  sinus congestion, backaches, headaches, depression, weight
  gain, chronic gastrointestinal troubles and fatigue.
  Chocolate, corn, wheat, dairy products, berries, eggs, yeast,
  shellfish, nuts and additives or preservatives are common
  offenders. To determine if you have a food allergy, keep a
  food journal, where you can compile a list of suspected
  foods and eliminate them one at a time for two to six weeks
  to identify culprit foods. Asthmatics should also avoid foods
  that cause heartburn since gastroesophageal reflux disease
  (GERD), commonly called acid reflux, has also been linked
  to asthma in some patients. A link between asthma and irritable bowel syndrome is also being established.

• **Infection.** Asthma has been linked to infection by the following organisms: *Chlamydia pneumoniae, Mycoplasma pneumoniae,* and the adenovirus and syncytial virus (responsible
  for many respiratory infections). Syncytial virus in adults
  has been linked to adult asthma, and rhinovirus (which
  causes the common cold) has been found to agitate asthma
  in both adults and children. Almost half of asthma sufferers
  also have sinus abnormalities, and up to 30 percent have
  sinusitis.

• **Allergens.** As mentioned, some allergens have been found
  to trigger asthma—dust, mold, tobacco smoke, air pollution,

chemicals, pesticides, roaches and even some medications. Between 20 and 55 percent of asthma sufferers have aspirin-induced asthma, meaning that symptoms are more severe after they take aspirin, ibuprofen or another nonsteroidal anti-inflammatory drugs (NSAIDs). These drugs are meant to reduce inflammation but seem to have the opposite effect on asthma inflammation. This type of asthma attack occurs more often after the patient has had a viral infection. If you suspect an allergen may trigger an attack, try to pinpoint what it might be and avoid it. Your doctor may be able to help you with this.

• **Hormones.** Hormone level changes in women have been found to affect the severity of asthma. Between 30 and 40 percent of asthmatic women experience fluctuations in asthma attacks related to their menstrual cycle. Women most likely to be affected are those who are older and have had asthma for a long time. Severe asthma attacks in these women are most likely to occur shortly before or after the start of their periods. Some doctors recommend birth control pills for these women. Pregnancy and menopause may also affect the severity and frequency of asthma attacks.

How Is Asthma Normally Treated?

Asthma sufferers can reduce the number of asthma attacks they experience by avoiding triggers like allergens, stress and certain environmental conditions; taking preventative drugs like anti-inflammatories and corticosteroids in the form of shots, pills and inhalers; and by drinking plenty of water and using humidifiers. Aerobic exercise like swimming may also be helpful, but asthmatics have to take extra precautions to avoid an exercise-induced attack. During an attack, individuals may be treated with adrenaline shots (epinephrine).

Many asthmatics are also using complementary medicine for asthma management. Acupuncture, aromatherapy and

Chinese medicine may be helpful, as can supplements like elecampane and mullein. Noni may also be very beneficial.

Noni and Asthma

If you remember, noni has been used to treat allergies. Its application for allergies has been largely unexplored by traditional medical research, but is based on noni's effects on malfunctioning cells and on the immune system. Its ability to normalize immunity is probably linked to its value as an allergy treatment. Anecdotal evidence supports noni supplementation for allergies. Those suffering from allergy-related asthma may find that noni reduces the number of asthma attacks an individual experiences. Noni's normalizing effect on cells may also have a positive effect on hormone levels, thereby decreasing the severity of attacks in affected women. Noni's antimicrobial properties may also reduce the number and severity of infections in vulnerable people.

DIABETES

Diabetes is the seventh leading cause of death (sixth-leading cause of death by disease) in the United States. It is estimated that there are nearly sixteen million Americans in the United States with diabetes, and approximately five million don't know it. A staggering 2,200 cases of this chronic, incurable disease are diagnosed each day. Even more disturbing, diabetes is the leading cause of adult blindness and kidney disease, and accounts for more than 75,000 deaths from heart disease each year. Diabetics are two to four times more likely to develop heart disease or suffer a stroke than healthy individuals, and nearly 70 percent of diabetics have some form of nerve damage, which can eventually lead to lower limb amputations. Leg amputation risk alone is fifteen to forty times higher for diabetics, and more than 50,000 diabetic amputations are performed every year, making it the largest cause of (non-traumatic) limb amputations in the United States.

Symptoms of diabetes include low energy, increased thirst and hunger, frequent urination and weight loss. Other symptoms include vision problems, circulation problems, an increased number of infections, nausea, impotence, mood changes and even nerve damage.

Unfortunately, those Americans who develop type-1 diabetes can do nothing to prevent it. It is true, however, that a growing number of individuals are being diagnosed with a more preventable form, type-2 diabetes. Experts link the increased incidence of type-2 diabetes with the the rise in obesity (and other factors), especially in children. However, diabetes can be successfully managed and, in some cases, prevented altogether. Let's take a quick look at what diabetes is, the risk factors for developing the disease, and how it can be treated.

What Is Diabetes and Who Is at Risk?

Diabetes is a blood sugar disease that affects the way your body processes and uses food. The whole problem stems from a substance that regulates blood sugar called insulin, the chemical messenger produced by the pancreas that links cells with the energy they need. Your body converts what you eat (specifically carbohydrates) into energy your cells can use (a simple sugar called glucose). Insulin is there to tell the cells (by linking to cell receptors) when glucose is available; cells cannot use glucose without the help of insulin. Blood sugar fluctuates in response to insulin—as insulin is released and glucose is metabolized by the cells, blood sugar drops. Another substance secreted by the pancreas raises blood sugar, and together they work to regulate blood sugar levels and keep them healthy.

Diabetes occurs when the pancreas stops producing insulin or insulin cells are attacked by the body's own immune system preventing proper glucose metabolism (type-1 diabetes). In the case of type-2 diabetes, the body stops producing enough insulin or cell receptors become resistant to insulin and the body cannot metabolize blood glucose properly. Some diabetics show signs of both contributing factors. Both types can lead to dangerously high blood sugar levels, but type-2 accounts for nearly *95 percent* of all cases of the disease.

The incidence of type-2 (or adult-onset) diabetes is on the rise due to factors such as sedentary lifestyles and obesity. Other risk factors for type-2 diabetes include age (individuals over forty-five have a higher risk of developing diabetes), pregnancy (especially with babies over nine pounds), a family history of diabetes, and members of minority groups such as African Americans, Latinos, Native Americans, Asian Americans and Pacific Islanders. Type-1 diabetes usually manifests itself during a person's childhood or teen years and affects Caucasians more than any other race.

Noni for Diabetics

In addition to the normal treatments for diabetes—insulin, drugs to mediate blood sugar, exercise and diet—many individuals are turning to CAM treatments. Individuals who suffer from "brittle diabetes" (frequent, unhealthy blood sugar fluctuations that are resistant to treatment) and those at risk for developing type-2 diabetes are often interested in complementary therapies because they offer what conventional medicine hasn't yet. Supplements such as chromium picolinate, zinc, magnesium, *Gymnema sylvestre*, bilberry and pycnogenol may be useful in lowering blood sugar naturally, and noni also has a long history of use for the disease.

Used historically in Hawaii and Tahiti to treat blood sugar abnormalities, noni is also the subject of diabetes-related university studies out of Nigeria. One 1999 study in the *Journal of Pharmacology* showed that a leaf extract of a close relative of noni, *Morinda lucida*, had significant hypoglycemic activity in

"My blood sugar levels are starting to stabilize"

"April 1, 1959, at the age of 15, I was diagnosed with insulin-dependent diabetes. Forty-three years later I praise God that I am still alive.

The diabetes quickly turned to a "brittle" type, meaning that I am extremely sensitive to insulin, especially fast-acting insulin. As the years go by, I have become extremely tired, experience stiffness and pain in my joints, and started experiencing high blood pressure.

My prayers were for balance in my life and to keep my energy levels up and the blood sugar in a good range of 120.

Last year (2001), three different people suggested that I take Tahitian noni juice for my diabetes. I was extremely skeptical about taking a fruit juice, let alone one from Tahiti! My research began and all reports were excellent, much to my surprise.

Three weeks ago, a fourth person, a very dear friend, called and said he was coming to visit and that he was bringing noni!

I started my regimen the very next day of one ounce in the morning and one ounce in the evening. The following day, I realized that I had no evidence of stiffness or pain in my left leg!

That first week, I realized an increase in my energy levels. My pains and aches disappeared; for example, I could now make tight fists and my shoulders no longer ached after sleeping on my side through the night. My blood sugar levels are starting to stabilize. I am now awaiting what the next blood test will show regarding my kidneys . . . Praise God!"

Gail E. Springer, USA

diabetic tests. The glucose-lowering compounds found in this plant are believed to have a similar composition to those in noni leaves, which would explain noni's traditional use for blood sugar disorders.

Noni also contains B-sitosterol, a proven blood sugar lowering compound. In laboratory tests, it was able to increase insulin levels (which lowered glucose levels). By doing so, B-sitosterol offered protection from ill effects of sustained high blood sugar. Noni's effects on xeronine levels may also help prevent cell malfunctions in the pancreas and the immune system that may lead to diabetes. Furthermore, its adaptogenic qualities and fiber content contribute to its ability to help stabilize blood sugar.

Kidney Disease

Each year about 80,000 individuals in the United States are diagnosed with kidney failure. Nearly 40 percent of these cases are the result of diabetes, but high blood pressure, heart disease and lupus have also been linked to the disease. Repeated bladder or kidney infections may also be contributing factors. Symptoms of kidney disease include increased thirst and urination, swelling of the hands and feet, loss of appetite, pale skin, fatigue, itchiness and an unpleasant taste in the mouth.

The kidneys are essential for proper waste removal in the body, and they also help regulate various body chemicals and blood pressure. When the kidneys become diseased (gradually or suddenly), they can become impaired and may even stop working altogether—a potentially deadly condition. When this happens, the body has no way to dispose of toxic waste products and slowly poisons itself. In this situation, a person has to be put on dialysis (a filtering therapy that replaces some kidney function) or receive a kidney transplant in order to survive.

While medical treatments can slow the progression of the disease, the best way to deal with this incurable condition is not to deal with it at all. Prevention is always preferred. Noni supplementation may reduce many risk factors for the disease, including high blood pressure, diabetes and heart disease, and its antibacterial power may prevent serious infection of the kidneys or urinary tract. Combined with a healthy lifestyle, a proper diet and drinking plenty of water, noni will increase your chances of avoiding this fatal disease. Noni is not recommended for patients with end-stage renal failure. For more information on kidney disease contact the National Kidney and Urologic Disease Information Clearinghouse at **nkudic@info.niddk.nih.gov** or visit their website at **www.niddk.nih.gov.**

DIGESTIVE PROBLEMS

According to the National Digestive Diseases Information Clearinghouse, nearly seventy million people are affected by digestive diseases, accounting for 13 percent of hospitalizations and fifty million visits to the doctor's office each year. Digestive diseases also cause thousands of deaths each year, contribute to 1.4 million disability cases and, according to statistics from the early nineties, cost the U.S. over one hundred billion dollars a year in direct (i.e. medical costs) and indirect (i.e. disability costs) expenses. Let's look at some of the most common digestive complaints and how noni may help.

Diarrhea

Diarrhea can be caused by a number of conditions, some benign while others may be very serious. Possible causes include stress, eating too much fiber or fruit, medications like antibiotics, irritable bowel syndrome, malabsorption, thyroid problems, lactose intolerance, diabetes, food poisoning, microbe infection, colitis, diverticulitis and even cancer. Diarrhea prompts over ten million doctor visits, and over five million prescriptions written to treat it each year. Of course, any abnormal or chronic cases of diarrhea should be reported to your healthcare provider. However, supplementing with noni may be helpful for diarrhea caused by stress, microbes, food poisoning and irritable bowel syndrome. Diabetics and cancer patients with chronic diarrhea may also find some relief with noni supplementation, though they should speak with a doctor before beginning a noni program. Not only can noni's proxeronine aid in proper intestine and colon function, its antimicrobial properties may help relieve diarrhea caused by a virus or bacteria.

Irritable Bowel Syndrome

Irritable bowel syndrome or IBS is the most common digestive disorder, affecting over five million people and disabling 400,000 of them. Sufferers are plagued with repeated bouts of constipation and diarrhea that occurs shortly after they eat, and symptoms can last for months. Individuals with IBS usually complain of cramping, bloating and increased gas. Some develop colitis, Crohn's disease or even cancer.

More women than men suffer with IBS, but many sufferers remain unaware that they have IBS. Symptoms often develop in a person's early to mid twenties and can be brought on by periods of extreme stress. In fact, about 10 to 15 percent of the U.S. adult population can expect to deal with at least one bout of irritable bowel syndrome. Researchers have also linked IBS to lactose intolerance, binge eating, smoking, antibiotics, antacids, antidepressants, sedatives and even sugar substitutes like aspartame.

Traditional treatment for IBS includes limiting dietary fat and animal products and increasing fiber and vegetable intake. Exercise and stress management classes are also recommended. Sufferers should also drink plenty of water. Supplements like psyllium, marshmallow, slippery elm and peppermint may also be helpful. Anecdotal evidence on noni reveals its therapeutic potential in this and related conditions as well.

Constipation

Constipation afflicts more than four million Americans, and it is the cause of over two million doctor visits and one million prescriptions each year. Surprisingly enough, serious constipation can lead to disability and even death. Experts say you should eliminate between once every three days to three times a day, depending on your age, diet and level of activity. Going longer than three days is considered unhealthy. Stools that are hard to pass may also signal a problem.

Women and the elderly are most likely to suffer from constipation, but anyone who consumes very little fiber, does not engage in regular exercise, or takes medications such as codeine, antacids, antidepressants, diuretics, medications for high blood pressure and even antihistamines regularly is at risk for chronic constipation.

Along with senna, cascara sagrada, buckthorn and psyllium, noni has been an effective treatment for constipation in some people. Several components of noni are thought to be responsible. Individuals taking noni for high blood pressure instead of prescriptions can avoid the constipation that is typically caused by medications for hypertension. Individuals taking noni for increased energy may become more active, and exercising is a great way to stay regular. More importantly, noni contains both soluble and insoluble fiber. That combined with its normalizing effect on the cells of the digestive tract help to promote good peristalsis in the bowel. Dietary fiber is one of the best treatments for occasional and chronic constipation, and may also be useful in the treatment of heart disease, obesity and diabetes. Of course, if you have been constipated for more than two weeks or if there is blood in your stool, see a doctor immediately.

Ulcers

If you regularly suffer from burning abdominal pain, especially in the morning or between meals, or after consuming citrus fruits, coffee or aspirin, you may be one out of every ten Americans who have an ulcer. Ulcer discomfort is often relieved by taking antacids and may cause black or bloody stool. Peptic (stomach) ulcers are basically breaks in the stomach lining, the esophagus or small intestine. Ulcers can lead to more serious problems in the pancreas, or cause anemia or even stomach cancer. Though relatively easy to treat, the true cause of ulcers is still the subject of debate. Stress, fast or fatty foods, tobacco, caffeine and alcohol abuse have all been blamed. The "Type A personality" theory was popular during the 1980s, but now scientists know that many factors can contribute to the formation of ulcers, including the overuse of aspirin or ibuprofen and the bacterium *Helicobacter pylori*.

Ulcers are traditionally treated with antibiotics and antacids. For more serious cases, surgery may be required. Noni's antibacterial constituents make it a good choice for ulcers that are caused by bacteria. Using noni for pain management may reduce the risk of ulcers caused by analgesics like aspirin. Noni may also help individuals quit smoking and consuming alcohol, both of which aggravate ulcers.

Indigestion

Indigestion is an all-inclusive word used to collectively describe a slew of problems, including flatulence, heartburn, abdominal discomfort, nausea or vomiting and general stomach upset. Any time normal digestion is interrupted, indigestion occurs. Occasional bouts of indigestion are unavoidable. If, however, it happens on a daily basis, steps should be taken to limit its impact. Chronic indigestion can be a sign that something more serious is going on, including stomach ulcers, cancer or gallstones.

The causes of indigestion are as numerous as the symptoms and include stress, improper diet and eating habits, smoking, obesity and microbial infection. Treatments for indigestion may be as simple as a dose of the pink stuff or much more elaborate—even including surgery if the problem is structural.

Depending on the cause, various CAM treatments may also be useful—acupressure, Ayurvedic medicine, slippery elm, ginger, chamomile, peppermint and digestive enzymes can all facilitate better digestion. Noni tackles indigestion by fighting possible infection, providing fiber for better elimination and by supplying a well balanced array of vitamins and mineral. Its healing properties may also protect the mucous membranes of the intestinal tract. When combined with regular exercise and a healthy diet, noni can minimize the effects and frequency of gastric upset in all its forms.

PAIN

One long-standing use for noni is treating acute and chronic pain. Noni provides an effective alternative to traditional prescription and over-the-counter pain killers, which have countless side effects (especially when taken for extended periods of time). They can cause depression, kidney and liver damage, stomach upset, ulcers and fatigue to name a few. Plus, pain killers merely mask symptoms and do nothing to address the source of the pain. On the other hand, noni repairs damaged cells while relieving pain. A 1990 study found that extracts derived from noni root have the ability to kill pain in animal experiments. Interestingly, it was during this study that the natural sedative action of the root was also noted. Xeronine has also been described as a pain reliever.

Aches and pains may be a normal part of day-to-day living, but when discomfort interferes with or undermines your routine, it's time to take action. In fact, chronic pain is responsible for more cases of disability than heart disease and cancer cases combined, and it is one of the top reasons for doctor visits. More than 25 percent of Americans will experience some type of chronic pain every year.

Migraines, back pain, fibromyalgia, reproductive disorders, cancer, Crohn's disease, joint pain and carpal tunnel syndrome are all sources of chronic pain. Inactivity, stress and obesity may also be linked to chronic pain. Cancer and accident survivors and the elderly are also more likely to suffer from chronic pain. Some studies have also found links between migraines in women and hormone imbalances. Pain management can include drugs, relaxation exercises, meditation, physical therapy or acupuncture. Below are some of the most common causes of chronic pain:

Migraines

Migraine headaches cause severe and even disabling episodes of pain. Sufferers often experience nausea or vomiting, visual disturbances and extreme sensitivity to light and sound in addition to extreme head pain. Migraines can last for just a few hours or up to three days, depending on the severity of the attack. They can recur several times a week or only a few times a year.

Blood vessel constriction is believed to be at the root of migraine headaches, but scientists are still unsure of all the mechanisms involved in the condition. Some connections have been made between serotonin level fluctuations and migraine headaches; links have also been established between estrogen and migraines. Family history is a factor, and numerous elements can trigger an attack, including various foods, caffeine, specific scents, hormone fluctuations, stress and even a change in the seasons. Exercise, sex and extreme cold can also trigger a headache.

Prescription drugs are often used to treat migraines, but acupuncture, biofeedback and chiropractic treatments have also been used. Aromatherapy with lavender oil is another option, as well as using feverfew, magnesium and niacin. Noni may offer significant benefits for migraine management.

Noni's effect on xeronine seems to play a role in proper serotonin production and utilization by the body. Serotonin is a neurotransmitter that not only impacts pain, but is involved in migraine pain, fibromyalgia, depression, premenstrual syndrome and sleeping disorders. Actually, some migraine drugs work by mimicking serotonin, and low blood serotonin can be used to predict a migraine. In fact, even estrogen fluctuations (which have been blamed for migraines) influence serotonin levels, possibly triggering a migraine. Although there is no specific proof of the link between noni and serotonin, some researchers believe a correlation exists between the two. Its analgesic effect is also beneficial for reducing migraine discomfort.

Arthritis

The word "arthritis" is actually an umbrella term used to describe over one hundred different problems, including osteoarthritis, infectious arthritis, ankylosing spondylitis (spinal arthritis), gout, bone spurs, rheumatoid arthritis and even lupus (an inflammatory disease of the connective tissues). Arthritis means "joint inflammation" and sufferers of the disease experience swelling, redness and pain in various joints and surrounding tissues. Although arthritis is usually associated with the elderly, almost three out of every five victims are under the age of sixty-five. In fact, approximately forty-two million Americans are affected with some form of arthritis.

For some arthritic conditions like lupus and rheumatism, the causes are not completely known, although though theories of autoimmune disorders, microbial infection and severe stress have all been proposed. Osteoarthritis is believed to be the result of joint wear and tear over time, and infectious arthritis is caused by a joint infection following severe illnesses, such as Lyme disease or a staph infection.

Traditional treatments for arthritis include anti-inflammatory drugs, corticosteroids and (sometimes) antibiotics. Meditation, chiropractic therapy, acupuncture and supplement therapy are some CAM treatments used for various types of arthritis, and are combined with traditional medications.

Noni supplementation may be able to replace traditional pain medications (or reduce their dosages), especially in early stages of the disease. As mentioned, noni's effect on serotonin may partially explain its use for arthritic pain. Noni also exerts positive effects on the immune system and is an effective antimicrobial.

One other link to arthritic pain may be the inability to properly digest proteins. Consequently, they can form crystal-like deposits which can lodge in joints. The ability of noni to enhance proper digestion through enhanced enzymatic function may help eliminate this particular type of arthritis. Moreover, the high alkaloid content of noni may be linked to its apparent anti-inflammatory action. Plant sterols found in noni help calm the inflammatory response which is what causes swelling and pain. In addition, the antioxidant effect of noni helps to decrease free radical damage in joint cells. These dangerous molecules can exacerbate discomfort and degeneration.

Although not all arthritic conditions will be relieved or reversed with noni, for those conditions caused by infection or autoimmune disorders, noni may be effective. Its cell-repairing properties may aid in overall joint repair, and taking noni before you suffer from any joint problems may help you avoid them altogether.

Back Pain

Almost half of the world's adult population suffers from back pain that lasts for a minimum of twenty-four hours and occurs at least once a year. That percentage is even higher for adults in the United States (near 80 percent). For a vast majority of these sufferers, the pain is not passing, but rather a chronic problem that persists on a monthly, weekly, or even daily basis. Back problems can be difficult to accurately diagnose and treat. Causes are varied—backstrain, osteoarthritis, spinal misalignment, pinched nerves, osteoporosis, a herniated disk, and even a kidney infection, menstrual cramps or a tumor.

Many experts blame a lack of exercise, stress, excess weight, anxiety and poor posture for chronic back problems that cannot be traced back to a physical problem in the spine itself. A number of health professionals believe that any back pain that can be relieved by massage therapy, relaxation techniques or physical therapy is most likely the result of muscle strain, not damage to the spine. If you have chronic undiagnosed back pain that is not caused by spinal injury, infection or cancer, noni may be helpful—directly and indirectly—for both treatment and prevention. Not only does noni have documented pain-relieving properties, it also boosts immune function, energy levels and resiliency against daily stressors. Noni users who have reported back pain relief usually experience other beneficial effects, like increased energy, which prompts more activity, thereby helping maintain or achieve an ideal weight. Noni users are giving their body systems the right mix of bioactive compounds that help achieve optimal levels of health and disease resistance. When noni therapy is combined with a beneficial diet and exercise program, the results are even better. Make sure to consult your doctor for specific stretching exercising designed to strengthen back muscles.

Fibromyalgia

Noni may be useful in the treatment of fibromyalgia due to its energy-boosting effects and pain-relieving properties. Fibromyalgia is characterized by depression, sleep disorders and ever-present fatigue, as well as chronic pain in specific places called tender (or trigger) points. The medical community knows relatively little about what causes fibromyalgia or how to cure it, yet millions of Americans have been diagnosed with the disease.

Traditional treatments usually include antidepressants,

sleeping pills and pain medication; however, noni may offer new hope to suffers because of natural analgesic properties and its positive effects on pain and fatigue. Moreover, some experts believe fibromylagia stems from a type of immune malfunction, and noni helps to normalize the immune system.

Research on the damnacanthal in noni fruit found it was able to inhibit the Epstein-Barr virus. There are established links between this virus and diseases like chronic fatigue syndrome (also linked to fibromyalgia). Noni's extraordinary immune-enhancing properties may prove helpful against these weaknesses. Furthermore, some experts theorize that neurotransmitter abnormalities may be at the root of fibromyalgia. Noni's cell normalizing effects may be able to repair these abnormalities. Anecdotal evidence also supports using noni for fibromyalgia.

Now that we know a little more about what noni can be used for and how it works on various conditions, lets take a closer look at how to use noni, the available forms of noni, side effects of supplementation, safety issues and dosage advice.

CHAPTER NINE

A Primer on Using Noni in All Its Forms

- Product preparation: a key to potency
- Available forms of noni
- Noni for pets
- Dosage advice
- Side effects
- Safety issues

- Twenty ways to use noni
- Noni use by part
- Combining noni with other agents
- Conclusion: using noni in your whole-health strategy

Now that you know what noni is, how it works and what it is used for, let's turn our attention to the specifics of using noni for health. If you have been using noni or would like to start, you may be wondering what form of noni to take, what brand of noni is best, or how much will work for your particular health problem. You may be concerned about combining noni with other medical treatments, or if noni is safe for pregnant and lactating women. This chapter is designed to answer all questions and concerns about using noni products, whether you are taking them internally or using them topically. I will discuss noni forms, dosage and safety as well as a number of ways in which noni can be used—including information on how noni may benefit your pets.

PRODUCT PREPARATION: A KEY TO POTENCY

One of the most important things to remember about using noni is that not all noni products are created equal. If you want an effective noni product, you may need to do a little research to find the right manufacturer. When buying noni products, look for reliable companies who will stand by their product's purity. Make sure they have research and development departments that can be contacted regarding proper aging and other processing techniques. The **Resource Guide** in the back of this book is a good place to start.

Here are some questions to ask companies when deciding whether to buy a noni product:

- Was the noni grown in an unpolluted, tropical environment?
- Who harvested the noni? Were local people involved who know how to properly harvest noni?
- How pure is the product? What processes does the noni undergo before it is packaged? What additives are in the noni product?
- How fresh in the noni when it is processed and packaged?

Harvesting Methods and Noni Purity

Harvesting methods, as discussed in **Chapter 2**, affect noni's quality and subsequent therapeutic effectiveness. The fruit needs to be picked at a certain stage of ripeness for the best benefit. The process by which it is cultivated and processed also affects its effectiveness. If you are using a supplement that contains other parts of the noni plant, the processing and combining of those constituents can also affect purity and the overall effect of the supplement.

AVAILABLE FORMS OF NONI

Although noni fruit is most commonly used, the leaves, root, bark, seeds and flowers of the noni plant also have health benefits. Several scientific studies on noni have explored the therapeutic benefits of all parts of the plant, not just the fruit. Some of you may be wondering if it is better to take one part of the noni plant or a combination. I believe that it may be more effective to take a combination of juice, root and leaf extracts for maximum effect, especially if treating a chronic condition. Noni can be purchased as leaf tablets, fruit juice, teas made from the leaf, freeze-dried fruit concentrates, capsulated juice extracts, chewable tablets, and oil. Leaf products are available in cold-pressed tablets and are sometimes included with other noni plant constituents, which contain a percentage of the fruit, bark, root and seeds for their individual therapeutic properties.

Shelf Life

Most noni products will last between one to two years if packaged and stored correctly. Always refrigerate juice products after opening and keep other products in a cool, dark and dry location.

Noni Leaf Teas

Teas have an advantage in that they contain a natural blend of whatever plant or plant parts used. Hot water releases therapeutic compounds found in the noni leaf, which after drinking, are quickly assimilated into the bloodstream. Teas made of leaf or bark constituents need a longer steeping time than regular tea—at least ten minutes to ensure that the desired plant properties infuse into the water. Using a porcelain cup is best. One advantage of teas in that you can control concentration with steeping time and tea bag quantity. Another marvelous advantage of noni leaf tea bags is that they can be used as mini poultices and placed directly on cuts, burns, bug bites, etc.

Water-Based Sprays

Like teas that are water-extracted, water-based concentrated sprays can directly target inflamed areas topically or be applied directly to the tongue for absorption. Sprays also have an advantage in that they can be used to make compresses, eyewashes, nasal irrigations and gargles.

Cold-Pressed Tablets

Cold-pressed tablets and encapsulated noni leaf parts (with no fillers) provide leaf parts in a more convenient form and can be more concentrated, which is ideal when fighting chronic diseases. Having the leaf in chewable form is also excellent for children or older individuals who may not be able to swallow tablets. Chewable tablets can also be pulverized and added to juices, soups and other liquids.

Noni Fruit Juice

Taking noni fruit in juice forms provides a complete and natural delivery system to the body with a synergistic and balanced array of enzymes and nutrients in their original form. As stated, noni fruit juice is the most popular way to take noni. In fact, many companies that sell noni only sell it in fruit juice form. A majority of the studies about noni deal with the therapeutic applications of noni juice. However, the whole noni plant has therapeutic benefit and different parts of the plant are used for different ailments, as discussed in **Chapter 2**. Parts can be used alone or in combination for the best effect.

NONI FOR PETS

Noni extracts are also excellent for pets and can be used to treat a variety of disorders. In fact, the Animal Emergency Center in Kentucky has used noni to successfully treat thousands of animals after one of the center's veterinarians found it useful for treating illnesses in his own family.

The juice can be given at one to three ounces daily depending on the size of the animal. (Some professionals recommend equating the animal's weight to that of a human, thereby determining if the animal should receive an adult or child's dose.) Leaf supplements or leaves from opened tea bags can be added to pet food. Noni leaf tea bags can be opened and leaf parts can be given directly to pets. Chewable tablets can also be pulverized and added to dog food or liquids administered with an eyedropper. Some dogs will readily eat the leaf just as they chew on grass during times of illness.

Noni can be used in animals for infection, worms, pain and inflammation, cancer and neurological problems.

DOSAGE ADVICE

When and how you take noni, as well as the form you take and the amount, can affect its effectiveness depending on what you are trying to accomplish with your noni treatment. Finding the right supplement and dosage for you may take some experimenting, but there are general guidelines for taking noni that will help you get the most out of it. This section will answer questions you have about who should take noni, what form you should take, how much or how long you can use noni and information on safely combining noni treatment with other supplements or prescriptions. I have also included suggestions for how noni can be used for a variety of health problems.

Suggested Use

Take noni supplements without food, coffee, nicotine or alcohol. Because of the juice's strong taste, however, you may

"My Lhasa apso was diagnosed with gastritis"

"In May of 1999 my seven-year-old Lhasa apso, Cleo, was diagnosed with severe Crohn's disease and gastritis. She was placed on a special diet along with four different medications. She required Predisone every day otherwise she was unable to eat and had loose mucoid stools.

In March of 2000, Cleo wasn't progressing and continued to have problems. Her internal medicine specialist suggested Cleo have a repeat colonoscopy and endoscopy. That is when I decided to look at nutritional healing as an alternative. Fortunately, I was referred to someone who immediately delivered a bottle of noni juice to us. My initial response was, "Dogs don't drink juice!" until I observed her lapping up a half teaspoon.

Presently, Cleo has been drinking noni juice for seven months (three teaspoons/ three times per day) and taking no medications. Cleo may never be totally without some problems, but she remains comfortable. Her appetite is excellent and her energy level is improved. A few months ago, her groomer commented on the fact that her coat appeared healthier. Occasionally, Cleo has a poor day and that is when I syringe a teaspoon or two into her mouth, and within a few minutes, she behaves as though she feels much better."

Anita H., USA

want to dilute it into cranberry or grape juice to make it more palatable. If you can't handle the taste or want a supplement that contains other parts of the noni plant or plant extracts, look for cold-pressed tablets or gel caps. These forms are convenient and should be taken according to label directions.

Before starting noni, test your response to your chosen noni product for at least five days by taking a reduced amount (approximately one tablespoon of juice a day for adults and one teaspoon for children, elderly and pregnant or nursing women). Any allergies/problems should emerge during this time.

Below are answers to frequently asked questions about using noni:

When (and how often) should I take noni?

Noni can be taken on a daily basis. Ideally, noni juice should be taken on an empty stomach prior to meals in divided doses (such as before breakfast and before dinner). The process of digesting food can interfere with the medicinal value of the alkaloid compounds found in noni.

How long will it take before I see results?

Some people feel the effects of noni within weeks (or even days), but in general, you should start to feel a difference after about two to three months, depending on the type and severity of your condition. If you have been taking noni for three months and still experience no change in your level of health, consider increasing your noni dosage. Also, make sure that the illness you are treating can in fact be treated by taking noni. Noni can't "cure" every health problem.

How long can I use noni?

If you experience no allergies or other side effects, you may take noni every day. Historical use suggests that noni can be taken for years (in reasonable dosages) without negative effects. To date, there are no known problems with taking noni long-term.

How much noni is enough?

The amount of noni you should take will vary depending on how you are using it, what form of noni you are taking and what you are taking it for. I will give some general guidelines, but you will probably have to experiment with different dosages until you find the optimal dosage amount for you. Dosages also vary according to the age of the user, their fitness level and weight. (Individuals over 250 pounds should increase recommended noni dosage by about one-half ounce for every fifty pounds over the 250 mark.)

Noni juice dosage recommendations usually fall between one-fourth of an ounce and two ounces daily. Healthy adults should usually take no more than one ounce daily, and children, no more than half an ounce to one ounce daily depending on their level of health and stomach sensitivity. Therapeutic treatment for serious or chronic illnesses (like HIV or cancer) may include much higher dosages (ten to twenty or more ounces per day), but those taking more than five ounces a day should definitely work with their doctor or other health professional.

The daily dosages of other products vary, and individuals taking these products should follow label instructions or seek the advice of a health professional who has worked with noni.

Can I take too much noni?

Although there is no known toxicity for noni juice, common sense suggests that any individual taking more than two to five ounces a day should seek the advice of a professional. Those taking supplements with various parts of the noni plant also need to take special care. Speak with the manufacturer of the product if you are wondering how much is too much and definitely consult with a doctor. If you experience side effects, decrease your dosage.

Serious health problems may require more noni, while healthy individuals may need very little noni for optimal health. Take as much noni as your body needs, not too much. Listen to your body. Some experts recommend that individuals with existing health problems, chronic conditions, serious illnesses or weakened immune systems initially "load" their body with noni by taking an increased amount for one to six months and then continue long-term noni supplementation at lower doses for maintenance and prevention.

Can I take noni if I am perfectly healthy?

Yes, you can. In fact, noni is an excellent preventive supplement. Of course, you will not need to take as much noni if you are in good health, and you will not need to take it as often. Many individuals using noni take it daily, but you may find that taking it every other day works fine for your needs.

Who shouldn't take noni?

Extracts of noni are considered safe if used as directed for most everyone; however, pregnant or nursing mothers should consult their physicians before taking noni or any supplement. Noni is safe for children and elderly individuals, but dosages may need to be altered. A few individuals may have an allergic reaction to noni, so test your response to noni by taking a reduced dose for at least five days before starting a full treatment program. Those with end-stage renal failure should also talk to their physician before taking noni.

I have to monitor my potassium intake—how much potassium does noni have?

Noni juice has less than half of the potassium of one orange, so you shouldn't experience any problems unless you are consuming large amounts of noni or if you have severe limits on how much potassium you are allowed daily.

SIDE EFFECTS

Any side effects reported by noni users have been considered minimal. Some of these include minor indigestion, allergic rash, or diarrhea. High doses of root extracts may cause constipation. If you experience any unwanted side effects, you may want to decrease your daily dosage.

A very small percentage of individuals may be allergic to noni (less than 2 percent of users, according to most reports).

If you develop hives, swelling, difficulty swallowing or severe diarrhea from taking noni, discontinue immediately. Some people who are initially (mildly) allergic to noni may overcome this sensitivity by halting noni supplementation for a week and then starting again with a reduced dose. Keep in mind that mild indigestion, itching or rashes that can accompany an allergy may be avoided by simply reducing your dose.

SAFETY ISSUES

Overall, noni is very safe to take. It has been included in the U.S. Dept. of Agriculture GRAS (Generally Regarded As Safe) listing since 1943. Extracts of noni are considered safe if used as directed; however, taking noni with coffee, alcohol or nicotine is not recommended. There are currently no substantiated, documented reports of serious negative reactions for noni other than a few individuals who were allergic to the plant. As mentioned, pregnant or nursing women, children and elderly individuals should take extra care when using noni. Also, those individuals using noni to treat serious conditions like diabetes, cancer or HIV, should check with their doctor for possible drug interactions or other contraindications.

TWENTY WAYS TO USE NONI

1. Soak a gauze bandage in a noni and water mixture and refrigerate for an effective headache compress.
2. To treat sore muscles, mix an equal amount of sesame oil and noni juice and gently massage into muscles.
3. A cotton ball soaked in noni juice or tea can be used to treat pimples, insect bites and even warts. It can also be applied to hemorrhoids or other skin irritations.
4. Replace your traditional antacid with a noni supplement.

Using Noni for Systemic Conditions

If you are using noni for systemic conditions like irritable bowel, candida, etc., you may experience temporary side effects. These side effects collectively are referred to as a *die-off effect*, and although they may seem negative, they are actually signs that the body is detoxifying itself of damaging waste products. You may feel ill at first, but symptoms will go away and afterward, you should feel dramatically better. Examples of cleansing reactions by the body include bloating and diarrhea, pimples, headaches, sweating, fatigue, joint pain, and rashes. Sometimes the die-off effect can be confused with allergies or other sensitivities to noni, which is why experts recommend first testing your reaction to noni by ingesting very small amounts before beginning full treatment. Also, anyone using noni for detoxification should make sure to drink plenty of purified water. To reduce extreme reactions, consider temporarily reducing your dosage, or begin noni treatment on a weekend, so you can take advantage of its detoxifying effects without having it interfere with your work schedule or weekday responsibilities.

5. Warm, sterilized noni tea or juice may be used in an eye-dropper to treat an ear infection.

6. Gargling with a noni mixture may relieve sore throat symptoms and treat the symptoms of gingivitis, as well as toothaches and bad breath. Canker sores may also be treated with noni mouthwash or a compress.

7. A diluted noni tincture may be used in nose drops to treat symptoms of sinusitis and allergies.

8. Adding noni to a sitz bath may relieve symptoms of yeast or bladder infections, postpartum pain and menstrual cramps.

9. Purified water and noni may be put in a spray bottle to relieve the discomfort of chicken pox, poison ivy, insect bites, sunburn, hives and other skin irritations.

10. Taking a noni tonic before surgeries, traveling and other potentially stressful events will boost your immune system, increase energy levels and help your body handle the extra stress.
11. Noni tea is a treatment for tonsillitis, colds and flu, and it may be beneficial for individuals with chronic fatigue, fibromyalgia, cancer and HIV.
12. The scent of noni seed oil may be used to reduce cravings, especially to nicotine, according to some experts.
13. Noni extract may be added to shampoo (or used to make your own shampoo) to treat dandruff and itchy scalp. It can also be used to get rid of head lice.
14. Back, hip and shoulder pain can be relieved by applying a large compress of cloth soaked in noni juice or other liquid noni mixture.
15. Include noni in your next detoxification program because of its cleansing and healing actions in the digestive system and its effects on the blood and the immune system.
16. Apply a warm washcloth soaked in noni juice or tea to skin to treat acne, rashes and dryness, or soak hands or feet in the noni liquid to treat joint pain, athlete's foot, blisters or even fungal infections. Noni soaks can help strengthen brittle nails, relieve the pain of ingrown nails and promote nail and cuticle health.
17. Noni can also be used for enemas or douches but should only be attempted with the supervision of your health care provider.
18. Mixing noni with clay may also be helpful for facials or for treating headaches and arthritic or rheumatic pain. It can also be used to treat carpal tunnel syndrome.
19. Noni can be made into a paste and directly applied to cuts, burns, insect stings and other skin wounds or infections.
20. Apply noni leaf extract directly to cuts to disinfect and stop bleeding.

NONI USES BY PART

Bark: digestive complaints, wounds, malaria, infant diarrhea, coughs, urinary disorders

Leaves: gout, gingivitis, eye infection, fever, regulating blood sugar, sore throat, prevent blood clotting, burns, boils, wounds, joints, ringworm, chest colds, cancer, regulating cholesterol levels, inflammation, viral and bacterial infections

Flowers: eye problems

Fruit: gum inflammation, throat problems, dysentery, blood poisoning, menstrual abnormalities, tuberculosis, arthritis, rheumatism, diabetes, regulating blood pressure, cardiovascular problems, ulcers, microbial infections, swollen tissue, wounds, boils, joint pain, acne, sores, staph infection, head lice, cell abnormalities, cancer

Root: fever, congestion, insomnia, gout, joint swelling, regulating blood pressure, intestinal parasites, pain, constipation, anxiety

COMBINING NONI WITH OTHER AGENTS

Noni supplements can be taken together with other medications and nutritional supplements although you should check with your doctor, especially those undergoing drug treatments for serious illness. Use caution, but since noni is a food supplement and not toxic, it is generally safe to use in conjunction with other treatments. In fact, in some cases it can even enhance the effectiveness of other treatments. However, don't decrease the dosage of any medication you may be taking without your physician's approval.

CONCLUSION: USING NONI IN YOUR WHOLE-HEALTH STRATEGY

Noni is not a miracle cure, nor is it the answer to every possible health problem. It is, however, a very promising botanical medicine that may offer additional options for successful healthcare, especially for those illnesses where conventional medicine fails to provide adequate treatment. When added to a comprehensive health strategy, which includes regular exercise, a proper diet and overall healthy living, noni's benefits are even more obvious.

As an investigative author, I have concluded that noni has more than enough credibility to justify its use in a complete personal protocol for improved health. Supplementation with noni appears to optimize health. When combined with regular exercise and healthy eating, I believe that health improvements can be dramatic. Noni supplementation should be a part of a life-long change in lifestyle and not a short-lived attempt at better health. Your chances for success will only increase with every healthy choice you make. Talk with your doctor, dietician or other healthcare professional for advice and support. Share your goals with your family and loved ones. Keep a diary of your habits, including your daily noni dosage amounts, and the results you experience. The more aware you are of your body, the more you will be able to give it what it needs. You may be surprised at the big results you get from even small changes. If there is one idea I would like to leave with you after reading this book, it is this: Noni has become part of an overall health revolution instigated by people who want to explore all their options for maximum wellness. Taking responsibility for your health is an empowering experience and staying informed is the key to a healthier and happier life.

Resource Guide

NONI INFORMATION AND RESEARCH

International Noni Certification Council (INCC)
http://www.incc.org

The INCC is a non-profit organization "created to educate the public about the history, research and benefits of *Morinda citrifolia*, or noni." Their website provides scientific findings and anecdotal evidence about noni's health benefits. They can be contacted through email at info@incc.org.

Cancer Research Center of Hawaii: The Noni Study
http://www.hawaii.edu/crch/CenStudyNoni.htm

Scientific study on potential cancer benefits of noni. For more information about the study, you can also contact Clinical Research Nurse, Faith Inoshita, R.N., M.S., at (808) 586-2979.

PURCHASING NONI PRODUCTS

Body Systems Technology
408 Live Oaks Blvd.
Casselberry, FL 32707
Office: (407) 767-6977
http://bodysystemtechnology
  .com

ForMor International
496 Hwy. 64 E.
Conway, AR 72032
Toll Free: (888) 270-4793
Office: (501) 336-0077
Fax: (800) 750-8155
http://formorintl.com

Hawaiian Herbal Blessings
810 Kokomo Rd. #6
Haiku, Maui, Hawaii 96708
Toll Free: (888) 424-NONI
Office: (808) 575-7829
Fax: (808) 575-9680
http://www.hawaiian-noni-
works.com

Morinda, Inc.
5152 N. Edgewood Dr.,
Suite 100
Provo, UT 84604
Toll Free: (888) 386-6664
http://www.morinda.com

Only Natural, Inc.
31 Saratoga Blvd.
Island Park, NY 11558
Toll Free: (800) 866-2887
Office: (516) 897-7001
Fax: (516) 897-9332
http://onlynaturalinc.com

Royal Farms
50th E. 100 S., Suite 205
St. George, UT 84770
Office: (435) 628-6715
http://www.royalnoni.com

Matrix Health Products
9316 Wheatlands Rd., Suite A
Santee, CA 92071
Toll Free: (800) 736-5609
Office: (619) 448-7550
http://www.matrixhealth.com

Nutrican Nutritionals Ltd.
175 West Beaver Creek, Unit 19
Richmond Hill, Ontario
Canada, L4B 3M1
Office: (905) 882-7798
Fax: (905) 882-7707
E-mail: info@nutrican.com
http://www.nutrican.com

**Polynesian Natural Health
Products**
1030 Calle Cordillera, Suite 106
San Clemente, CA 92674
Toll Free: (877) POL-NONI (877-
765-6664)
Office: (949) 366-9857
Fax: (949) 366-9859
http://www.noni-source.com

Tahiti Products Inc.
5757 Wilshire Blvd., Suite 359
Los Angeles, CA 90036
Toll Free: (800) 796-2188
Office: (323) 525-0770
Fax: (323) 525-1773
http://www.puretahitinoni.com

Bibliography

Abbot, Isabella and Shimazu Colleen. "The Geographic Origin of the plants most commonly used for medicine by hawaiians." *Journal of Ethnopharmacology* (1985): 14, 214.

Agomo, P., et al. "Antimalarial medicinal plants and their impact on cell populations in various organs of mice." *African Journal of Medicine and Medical Sciences.* (1992 Dec): 21(2), 39–46.

Altonn, Helen. "Noni research will begin to test the plant against cancer and its symptoms." *Star Bulletin.* Honolulu, Hawaii. July 19, 2001.

"American Heart Association 2002 heart and stroke statistical update." American Heart Association. 2002.

"An eating plan for healthy Americans." American Heart Association. 2001.

Asuzu, I., et al. "Effects of *Morinda lucida* leaf extract on *Trypanosoma brucei* infection in mice" *Journal of Ethnopharmacology.* (1990 Oct):30(3), 307–13.

Yoshikawa, M., et al. "Chemical constituents of Chinese natural medicine, *Morindae radix*, the dried roots of *Morinda officinalis*, structures of morindolide and morofficinaloside" *Chemical and Pharmaceutical Bulletin.* (Tokyo) (1995 Sep):43(9), 1462–5.

Bryan, E. *Samoan and Scientific Names of Plants Found in Samoa.* Complied for the Governor of Samoa, Hamilton Library, University of Hawaii, 1935.

Bushnell, O., et al. "Antibacterial properties of some plants in Hawaii." *Pacific Science.* (1950): 4.

"Cancer Prevention and Early Detection Facts and Figures 2002." American Cancer Society. 2002.

Choi, Y., et al. "Induction of apoptosis by ursolic acid through activation of caspases and down-regulation of c-IAPs in human prostate epithelial cells." *International Journal of Oncology.* (2000 Sep):17(3), 565–71.

Dittmar Alexander "*Morinda citrifolia* L. use in indigenous Samoan medicine." *Journal of Herbs, Spices and Medicinal Plants.* (1993): 1(3), 89–91.

"Dr. Heinicke and the Secrets of Noni." *Health News.* Triple R. Publishing, 3(2), 4.

Elkins, Rita, M.H. *Polynesian Noni: Prize Herb of the South Pacific.* UT: Woodland Publishing, 2000.

Elkins, Rita, M.H. *The Pocket Herbal Reference.* UT: Woodland Publishing, 2002. Second edition.

Gupta, M., et al. "Anti-inflammatory and antipyretic activities of B-sitosterol." *Planta Medica.* (1980): 39, 157–163.

Heinicke, R. "The pharmacologically active ingredient of noni." University of Hawaii and R.M/ Heinicke. *Cell Regeneration: Unlocking the Secrets of Tahitian Noni.* (audio tape)

Hiramatsu, M., et al. "Induction of normal phenotypes in RAS-transformed cells by damnacanthal from *Morinda citrifolia.*" *Cancer Letters.* (1993): (73), 161–66.

Hirazumi, A., et al. "An immunomodulatory polysaccharide-rich substance from the fruit juice of *Morinda citrifolia* (noni) with antitumour activity." *Phytotherapy Research.* (1999 Aug): 13(5), 380–7.

Hirazumi, A., et al. "Anticancer activity of *Morinda citrifolia* on intraperiotneally implanted Lewis lung carcinoma in syngenic mice." *Proceedings of the Western Pharmacology Society.* (1994): (37), 145–46.

Hirazumi, A., et al. "Immunomodulation contributes to the anticancer activity of *Morinda citrifolia* (noni) fruit juice." *Proceedings of the Western Pharmacology Society.* (1996): 39, 7–9.

Hiwasa, T., et al. "Stimulation of ultraviolet-induced apoptosis of human fibroblast UVr-1 cells by tyrosine kinase inhibitors." *FEBS Letters.* (1999 Feb 12): 444(2–3), 173–6.

Hobbs, Christopher, L.Ac., A.H.G. "Adaptogens—Herbal Gems to Help Us Adapt." *HealthWorld Online.*

Ivorra, M., et al. "Antihyperglycemic and insulin-releasing effects of B-sitosterol." *3-B-D-Glucoside and Its Aglycone, B-Sitosterol.* Archives of the International Pharmacodyn. (1998): 296, 224–231.

Jacobson, B.H. and S.G. Aldana. "Relationship between frequency of aerobic activity and illness-related absenteeism in a large employee sample." *Journal of Occupational and Environmental Medicine.* (2001 Dec): 43(12), 1019–25.

Kim, D., et al. "Apoptotic activity of ursolic acid may correlate with the inhibition of initiation of DNA replication." *International Journal of Cancer.* (2000 Sep 1): 87(5), 629–36.

Leistner, E. "Isolation, identification and biosynthesis of anthraquinones in cell suspension cultures of *Morinda citrifolia.*" *Planta Medica.* (1975): Suppl, 214–24. (German.)

Levand, O. and H. Larson. "Some chemical constituents of *Morinda citrifolia.*" *Planta Medica.* (1979 June): 36(2), 186–7.

Liu, G., et al. "Two novel glycosides from the fruits of *Morinda citrifolia* (noni) inhibit AP-1 transactivation and cell transformation in the mouse epidermal JB6 cell line." *Cancer Research.* (2001 Aug): 1; 61(15), 5749–56.

Makinde, J. and P. Obih. "Screening of *Morinda lucida* leaf extract for antimalarial action on *Plasmodium berghei* in mice." *African Journal of Medicine and Medical Sciences.* (1985 Mar–Jun): 14(1–2), 59–63.

Morton, Julia. "The ocean-going noni or Indian mulberry (*Morinda citrifolia,* Rubiaceae) and some of its colorful relatives." *Economic Botany.* (1992): 46(3), 243.

Mueller, BA., et al. "Noni juice (*Morinda citrifolia*): hidden potential for hyperkalemia?" *American Journal of Kidney Disorders.* (2000): 35(2), 310–2.

Navarre, Isa. *76 Ways to Use Noni Fruit Juice for Better Health.* UT: Pride Publishing, 2001.

"Noni plant may help TB." *AIDS Patient Care Studies.* (2001 March): 15(3), 175.

Olajide, O., et al. "Evaluation of the anti-diabetic property of *Morinda lucida* leaves in streptozotocin-diabetic rats." *The Journal of Pharmacy and Pharmacology.* (1999 Nov): 51(11), 1321–4.

Peerzoda, N., et al. "Vitamin C and elemental composition of some bush-fruits." *Journal of Plant Nutrition.* (1990): 13(7), 787.

Pokrovskii, A., et al. "Immunomodulating activity of ursolic acid derivatives." *Doklady Akademii Nauk.* (1999 Nov): 369(3), 414–5.

Raj, R. "Screening of indigenous plants for anthelmintic action against human *Ascaris lumbricoides.*" *Indian Journal of Physiology and Pharmacology.* (1975 Jan–Mar): 19(1).

Sittie, A., et al. "Structure-activity studies: in vitro antileishmanial and anti-malarial activities of anthraquinones from *Morinda lucida.*" [letter] *Planta Medica.* (1999 Apr): 65(3), 259–61.

Solomon, Neil, M.D., Ph.D. *The Noni Phenomenon.* UT: Direct Source Publishing, 1999.

Solomon, Neil, M.D., Ph.D. *Tahitian Noni Juice: How Much, How Often, for What.* UT: Direct Source Publishing, 2000.

Subbaramaiah, K., et al. "Ursolic acid inhibits cyclooxygenase-2 transcription in human mammary epithelial cells." *Cancer Research.* (2000 May 1): 60(9), 2399–404.

Tona, L., et al. "Antiamoebic and phytochemical screening of some Congolese medicinal plants." *Journal of Ethnopharmacology.* (1998 May): 61(1), 57–65.

Tona, L., et al. "Antimalarial activity of 20 crude extracts from nine African medicinal plants used in Kinshasa, Congo." *Journal of Ethnopharmacology.* (1999 Dec 15): 68(1–3), 193–203.

Wang, M., et al. "Novel glycosides from noni (*Morinda citrifolia*)." *Journal of Natural Products.* (2000 Aug): 63(8), 1182–3.

Wang, M., et al. "Novel trisaccharide fatty acid ester identified from the fruits of *Morinda citrifolia* (noni)." *Journal of Agricultural and Food Chemistry.* (1999 Dec): 47(12), 4880–2.

Whistler, Arthur W. *Polynesian Herbal Medicine.* National Botanical Garden, Hong Kong: 1992.

Yan, H., et al. "Effect of moderate exercise on immune senescence in men." *European Jounral of Applied Physiology.* (2001 Dec): 86(2), 105–11.

Younos, C., et al. "Analgesic and behavioral effects of *Morinda citrifolia.*" *Planta Medica.* (1990): 56, 430–34.

Zenk, M., et al. "Anthraquinone production by cell suspension cultures of *Morinda citrifolia.*" *Planta Medica.* (1975): Suppl, 79–101.

Index

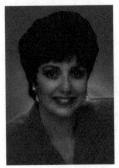

RITA ELKINS, M.H., has worked as an author and research specialist in the health field for the last ten years, and possesses a strong background in both conventional and alternative health therapies. She is the author of numerous books, including *Solving the Depression Puzzle*, which discusses the various options for effectively overcoming the complex problem of depression, *The Pocket Herbal Reference*, *The Complete Fiber Fact Book*, and *The Herbal Emergency Guide*. Rita has also authored dozens of booklets exploring the documented value of natural supplements like SAMe, noni, blue-green algae, chitosan, stevia and many more. She received an honorary Master Herbalist Degree from the College of Holistic Health and Healing in 1994.

Rita is frequently consulted for the formulation of herbal blends and has recently served on the 4-Life Research Medical Advisory Board. She is a regular contributor to *Let's Live* and *Great Life* magazines and is a frequent host on radio talk shows exploring natural health topics. She lectures nationwide on the science behind natural compounds and collaborates with medical doctors on various projects. Rita's publications and lectures have been used by companies like Nature's Sunshine, 4-Life Research, Enrich, NuSkin, and Nutraceutical to support the credibility of natural and integrative health therapies. She recently co-authored the award-winning *Soy Smart Health* with *New York Times'* best-selling author Neil Solomon, M.D.

Rita resides in Utah, is married, and has two daughters and two granddaughters.